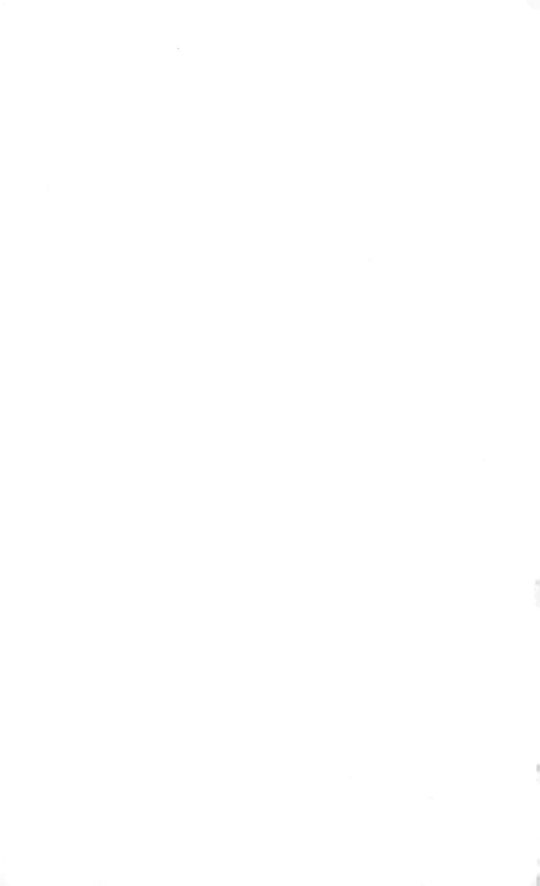

THE BEAUTY MOLECULE

THE
BEAUTY
MOLECULE

Introducing Neuroceuticals,
the Breakthrough for Ageless Beauty

NICHOLAS PERRICONE,
M.D., MACN

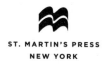

ST. MARTIN'S PRESS
NEW YORK

First published in the United States by St. Martin's Press, an imprint of St. Martin's Publishing Group

THE BEAUTY MOLECULE. Copyright © 2025 by Nicholas Perricone. All rights reserved. Printed in the United States of America. For information, address St. Martin's Publishing Group, 120 Broadway, New York, NY 10271.

www.stmartins.com

Credit for illustrations: Tata Bobokhidze

The Library of Congress Cataloging-in-Publication Data is available upon request.

ISBN 978-1-250-28679-6 (hardcover)
ISBN 978-1-250-28680-2 (ebook)

Our books may be purchased in bulk for promotional, educational, or business use. Please contact your local bookseller or the Macmillan Corporate and Premium Sales Department at 1-800-221-7945, extension 5442, or by email at MacmillanSpecialMarkets@macmillan.com.

First Edition: 2025

10 9 8 7 6 5 4 3 2 1

This book is dedicated to Jerry Weintraub,
whose exceptional talents, brilliance, wisdom, and kindness
are legendary. He was an enthusiastic supporter of my work,
and I am most honored to have known him as a great friend.

In Memoriam
Chim Potini, Harry, G. Preuss, M.D., Stephen Sinatra, M.D.

CONTENTS

INTRODUCTION

The Beauty Molecule: 10 Years in the Making

As I nursed a cup of green tea and read the news on the Internet, a 24-point headline from the United Kingdom's *Financial Times* caught my eye: "Scientists Discover the Secret of Aging." The article explained how one of the biggest puzzles in biology—how and why living cells age—had been solved by an international team based at the UK's Newcastle University. . . . The research . . . showed that when an aging cell detects serious DNA damage, which may be the result of general wear and tear from daily living, it sends out internal signals. These distress signals trigger the cells' mitochondria, the energy-producing part of the cell, to make free-radical molecules which instruct the cell either to destroy itself or to stop dividing. . . .

THE QUOTE YOU HAVE JUST read is an excerpt from chapter 1 of my past book *Forever Young*, published more than a decade ago. My own research has long shown that the scientific discovery described in the *Financial Times* is 100 percent accurate. Aging does indeed begin in the mitochondria, the all-important energy-producing part of the cell. This fact has been the focal point of my own research. I have identified what I call the Beauty Molecule, which protects and repairs the mitochondria to slow cellular aging. But it is not just the Beauty Molecule that makes this book so revolutionary. You will find the breakthrough secret to restoring the body's master antioxidant to youthful levels. This miraculous combination of amino acids—glycine and N-acetylcysteine—can repair the mitochondria and reverse many of the unwanted hallmarks of aging, ranging from a thickening waistline to insulin resistance to high blood pressure, just to name a few.

In these pages we will unlock an age-old secret of the natural world to discover the magic of pheromones. We tackle the question of whether a unique combination of pheromones and neuropeptides can change our lives, beginning with our most important relationships. We reveal the transformative effects of neuroceuticals, designed to transform both the skin and the brain in what can only be the essence of "smart beauty." Another new and revolutionary discovery in the world of weight loss is also shared for the first time. As new pharmaceuticals take the world by storm with daily stories of celebrities' dramatic weight loss, we offer a safe and effective alternative. Rather than injectables with potential for side effects, transdermal peptide solutions give us the results we have heretofore only dreamed of—safely and effectively. And could these same transdermal peptides in a cosmetic gel formulation rejuvenate our skin in ways beyond our wildest imagination? Read on to learn how these transformative discoveries are the inspiration for this book.

Though the correlation between inflammation and aging has only recently been recognized, I have spent my entire medical career studying this connection and searching for ways to subvert it. Today, research, academia, industry, and medicine all accept the causal relationship between inflammation and most chronic degenerative diseases, an astonishing list that includes arthritis, multiple sclerosis, atherosclerosis, diabetes, Alzheimer's, osteoporosis, cirrhosis, bowel disorders, cancer, stroke, and, of course, aging. There was not always tacit acceptance that inflammation, disease, and aging are connected. The theories I expressed in my books, including the claim that diet has a direct effect on the inflammatory response, were often ridiculed. I am pleased to say that these experts have since had to "eat" their words! In fact, metabolic dysfunction is the primary cause of chronic inflammation and disease.

I have been recognized as the "father of the nutrition-inflammation theory of aging" because inflammation has been the unifying theme of my books from the start. I revolutionized our view of aging by characterizing it as a treatable disease. Science has since agreed with this premise and recognized that chronic, low-level inflammation is the fundamental cause of aging and disease. Once that fact was accepted, I knew we were on our way to total physical, mental, and emotional rejuvenation.

Armed with this knowledge, I set about to find the root of inflammation. If I could discover the answer, I hoped to be able to provide an antidote or, because inflammation has more than one cause, multiple strategies to stop and reverse the deleterious effects. That is what I have spent the past 10 years doing.

During that time, I have often been asked by friends, colleagues, and readers why I have not written another book. I tell them there are two good reasons. Number one is that I would not publish a book unless I had something new to say. Second, I wanted to publish when a new generation would benefit from the discoveries that have been made.

The Wrinkle Cure, my first book, was groundbreaking. It was published just as baby boomers began to confront aging. This "youthquake" generation was facing a future in which they were no longer young. They were determined not to age like their parents. They demanded solutions. They wanted to know how to keep their bodies and minds as active and vital as they were in their teens and twenties. My book struck a chord, achieving almost instant bestseller status because I provided simple explanations and strategies for slowing down the aging process. The advice and suggestions on beauty and health I made then are still relevant and effective today. At the time, I was aware that a lot of what was being written had it wrong. False and incorrect information was everywhere. I was delighted to be able to set the record straight.

Now the day has arrived for a new book, *The Beauty Molecule*. Twenty years ago, *The Wrinkle Cure* set the stage for my subsequent bestsellers and the award-winning public television specials that followed. *The Beauty Molecule* raises what was promised in *The Wrinkle Cure* to a new level. My new book answers the question, Is there really a wrinkle cure? I can answer that not only is there a wrinkle cure, but I have also identified what I call the Beauty Molecule, a versatile neurotransmitter that protects the mitochondria.

The Beauty Molecule takes my initial premise to new heights. In the upcoming chapters, I will share breakthrough strategies designed to augment the production and actions of the Beauty Molecule. The result? A restored, radiant, youthful beauty; enhanced cognitive function; increased mental and physical energy; better regulation of your metabolism; and newfound serenity. We know now that the Beauty Molecule is central to the achievement of these goals. The Beauty Molecule's ability to repair the mitochondria is what makes it an agent of radiance, health, and longevity. I am excited to share these revelations with you. Please visit my website, PerriconeMD.com, for updates!

Nicholas Perricone, M.D., MACN

PART 1

THE BREAKTHROUGH DISCOVERY

1

INTRODUCING THE BEAUTY MOLECULE

AS I HAVE LONG TAUGHT, age-related damage to cells begins in the mitochondria, the energy portion of the cell, which is critical for health and longevity. Scientists now agree that the decline of the mitochondria results in aging on a cellular level. My decades-long quest has been to find the best strategies to protect and repair this vital part of the cell. The discovery of the Beauty Molecule expands and deepens my initial theories of inflammation. I have considered inflammation to be the final common pathway in aging and disease, and now we have discovered the key to turning off inflammation.

I have identified the multitasking neurotransmitter acetylcholine (ACh) as the Beauty Molecule, our first line of defense against aging. Looking for a way to fight inflammation, I found a powerful mediator to do that and more. The agent of radiance, health, and longevity, acetylcholine fights inflammation in several ways.

Acetylcholine has an important role in repairing damaged mitochondria and ridding the body of damaged, senescent cells. In addition to mitochondrial repair, acetylcholine functions in the central nervous system as an important neurotransmitter to enhance memory and cognition, which are unquestionably affected by aging. The Beauty Molecule is also the primary neurotransmitter of the parasympathetic nervous system, which, among other functions, turns off the inflammatory response.

The Beauty Molecule is also fundamental to movement. Motor activity is created by neurons that send a message to the muscles to stimulate contraction. The release of acetylcholine at the neuromuscular junction causes muscles to contract, creating movement.

The Beauty Molecule has another important function. ACh fights inflammation by inhibiting the inflammatory cascade set in motion by the immune system to protect the body against infectious disease and foreign invaders. The immune system consists of protective white blood cells called leukocytes and macrophages. The macrophages have receptors for the Beauty Molecule called alpha-7 nicotinic receptors because they can be activated by nicotine. Their key function is to trigger rapid neural and neuromuscular transmissions. When acetylcholine attaches to macrophages, the nicotinic receptors mediate and mitigate overreaction of the immune system by decreasing the production and release of pro-inflammatory cytokines, which prevents neuroinflammation.

As we age, our levels of acetylcholine decline, and muscle tone is reduced. Instead of staying short and tight, the muscles become elongated and relaxed, resulting in a sagging face and body. The way to improve muscle tone is to increase acetylcholine levels. A key component of this book is to show you what you can do to boost the levels of the Beauty Molecule in your body to revive youthful skin and muscle tone.

FIRST BRUSH WITH ACETYLCHOLINE

My first introduction to the effects of acetylcholine in a clinical setting occurred during my residency when I did my rotation in ophthalmology, which deals with the diagnosis and treatment of eye disorders. You may be wondering what the Beauty Molecule has to do with eye problems. As you will learn, there is not an area of the body that is not impacted by acetylcholine. The Beauty Molecule plays a vital role in all physical functions. Even the eye is affected by ACh, which helps to maintain rapid eye movement (REM) sleep, during which we dream.

I witnessed acetylcholine in action firsthand in the office of Dr. Frank Rosenbaum during my ophthalmology rotation. Dr. Rosenbaum asked me to do an interview and history on a patient whose chief complaint was a droopy eyelid. I examined the patient, took a history, and then discussed my findings with Dr. Rosenbaum.

One of the diseases that present with a symptom of drooping eyelid is myasthenia gravis, an autoimmune disease that attacks the receptors of the motor nerves, resulting in varying degrees of muscular weakness. The weakness can result in double vision, a drooping eyelid, difficulty speaking, and trouble walking. Myasthenia gravis is characterized by our immune cells attacking the acetylcholine receptor sites on the muscles, preventing them from responding to acetylcholine messages. When that happens, the muscles do not contract as they should, which is seen clinically as muscle weakness. With myasthenia gravis, the most commonly affected muscles are those of the eyes and face and those used for swallowing.

To determine the cause of the drooping eyelid, Dr. Rosenbaum explained that there was a 2-minute test utilizing a pharmaceutical called Tensilon. No longer recommended as a first-line test, it involved an injection of Tensilon, which can decrease the activity of acetylcholinesterase, an enzyme that breaks down acetylcholine. When the enzyme is inhibited, acetylcholine levels increase in the neuromuscular junction, resulting in increased muscle tone. If the eyelid did not open in response to the Tensilon injection, we could assume that myasthenia gravis was the problem. Nerves typically release ACh, which binds to acetylcholine receptors on muscles to activate them. If the drooping eyelid responded to the Tensilon, we could assume that myasthenia gravis could be blocking, inhibiting, or destroying acetylcholine in the neuromuscular junction.

I prepared the injection for the patient and explained to him what we were looking for. After the injection, the eyelid remained closed, meaning the Tensilon test was negative. We concluded that the problem was probably not myasthenia gravis.

This case illustrates the Beauty Molecule in action or absence. Myasthenia gravis causes the immune system to block or destroy acetylcholine receptors. When the muscles do not receive the ACh signal, they cannot function normally. Without acetylcholine, muscles cannot contract.

When it comes to the face, it is not wrinkles that are the greatest culprit in giving an aged appearance. It is the loss of anatomical position that results in the sagging and drooping of the underlying muscles. Anatomical position, also called standard anatomical position, refers to the specific body orientation used when describing an individual's anatomy. A clear and consistent way of describing human physiology is of importance in anatomy because it is the position of reference for anatomical nomenclature. The Beauty Molecule causes muscles to contract and tighten under the skin, enabling us to maintain a youthful appearance by maintaining our youthful anatomical position. For many years I have advocated the use of topical DMAE (dimethylaminoethanol), an organic compound that is a powerful anti-inflammatory. It is a precursor of choline, which increases production of acetylcholine and helps maintain a lifted, firmed, and toned appearance in both the face and body.

EATING TO BOOST ACETYLCHOLINE PRODUCTION

We can increase levels of acetylcholine through a variety of methods, such as diet, drugs, medications, and nutritional supplements. Certain foods, and supplements like DMAE, significantly influence the production of the Beauty Molecule. Foods that contain choline, an essential nutrient, boost the synthesis of acetylcholine. The main dietary sources of choline are animal-based products that are rich in choline—grass-fed beef, free-range poultry, fish, dairy products, and eggs. Cruciferous vegetables and certain beans also are rich in choline, as are nuts, seeds, and whole grains. Consuming these foods will boost your body's production of the Beauty Molecule.

CHOLINE-RICH FOODS TO BOOST PRODUCTION OF THE BEAUTY MOLECULE

You can boost acetylcholine by taking supplements that contain choline, but I always prefer the natural route. You can add to your choline intake with your choice of foods rich in choline, for example:

- Free-range chicken and turkey
- Cod
- Kidney beans
- Quinoa
- Grass-fed beef
- Shiitake mushrooms
- Almonds
- Cruciferous vegetables
- Quinoa

These foods not only fight inflammation but also protect and restore the mitochondria.

Another way you can indirectly increase acetylcholine levels is with supplements that function by inhibiting the enzyme acetylcholinesterase, making more of the Beauty Molecule available. Examples of these substances are ginkgo biloba and huperzine A.

Other foods have an adverse effect on levels of ACh and other critical neurotransmitters. Foods and beverages that are pro-inflammatory are the culprits. You will learn about these foods in the following chapter.

Eating to fight inflammation has been the foundation of my program for more than 20 years. In my dermatology practice, I routinely took a brief dietary history and explained the importance of the anti-inflammatory diet. When I treated patients with traditional medicine and medications, regardless of their condition or symptoms, they always did better when an anti-inflammatory diet was added. Skin radiance and tone are barometers of what is going on inside us. The most noticeable results of following an anti-inflammatory diet are radiant skin and increased contour line.

Before a review of the anti-inflammatory diet, the cornerstone of beauty, health, and longevity, I first want to explain how I came to my conclusions about increasing health span and longevity—about my inspiration, education, and, most important, my motivation.

2

BACK TO THE BEGINNING

MY FASCINATION WITH NUTRITION AND its powerful influence on physical and mental health was born shortly after my discharge from the US Army. I went to see an internal medicine doctor for a physical examination. Although I was declared perfectly healthy, I had been experiencing an almost debilitating fatigue. Only in my early twenties, I should have been bursting with energy, ready to take on the world and its exciting challenges. Instead I was mentally and physically exhausted. I also suffered from allergies.

In search of help, I read Linus Pauling's books and was intrigued by his theories about vitamin C and the common cold. I also read the work of Adelle Davis, a popular—if a bit radical—nutritionist of the 1960s and '70s. These two forward-thinking individuals taught me the critical importance of diet and dietary supplements in health and well-being. Desperate for answers, I eagerly followed their advice. As I experimented with various nutritional supplements and food choices, I started to feel more energetic.

I had been weight training since I was 15, and added to my stretching exercise in the morning. Regular exercise builds muscle, and I became more physically fit. I found that I was not only more productive but also more enthusiastic about my work and daily life. My allergies abated. My cognitive function and concentration improved greatly. I was thrilled to experience such unexpected changes.

FROM SHAKESPEARE TO STETHOSCOPE– THE ROAD TO MEDICAL SCHOOL

The first step in my post-army career was a position with a nonprofit organization, the Muscular Dystrophy Association, famous for its annual fundraising telethons hosted by Jerry Lewis. Muscular dystrophies are a genetically and clinically heterogeneous group of rare neuromuscular diseases. Over time the diseases cause progressive weakness and breakdown of skeletal muscles, affecting children who appear to be normal at birth but later become disabled.

Serving as director of the Philadelphia chapter, I was intimately involved in patient services. I got to know the children firsthand and witnessed the tragic progression of the disease. The experience sparked such a powerful interest in medicine that I started to think about going back to school.

Bruce McLucas, a young doctor in training at the Yale School of Medicine, who worked with us and the children at the Muscular Dystrophy Association, encouraged me to consider medicine because I was so knowledgeable about nutrition and its relationship to disease processes. Although intrigued by the idea, I was an English literature major. I did not have the science courses prerequisite for medical school. I wondered if I could make the transition from Shakespeare to stethoscope. Dr. McLucas explained that I needed only about eight courses in basic sciences, such as chemistry, organic chemistry, physics, and biology. That seemed doable to me.

I began to take courses in the evenings after work to achieve the core requirements for entry into medical school. I was surprised that I enjoyed the science courses. I also had to take the Medical College Admission Test (MCAT), a standardized, multiple-choice test that has been a part of the medical school admissions process for more than 90 years.

On the day of the test, as all of us waited to begin, I realized that the other aspiring medical school candidates were just as nervous as I was. As I took the test, I was relieved to find that my hard work and study had prepared me well. I began to believe that just maybe this journey was not hopeless.

When I received the test results, I was elated to learn I had done very well. I applied to five medical schools and was accepted by three of them. I had to look at the financial side of each medical school as well as the benefits and offerings. When I interviewed at the College of Human Medicine at Michigan State University, I was very interested. The medical school had a philosophy different from that of most medical schools. They taught the prospective physician to treat the individual and not the disease. This almost revolutionary concept resonated with me. During the interview, I had the feeling that Michigan State University would be the perfect place to pursue my future calling.

In medical school, the first 2 years are normally devoted to book learning. It is not until the second 2 years that students begin actual work with patients. However, in addition to the traditional methods of teaching, MSU offered students during their first 2 years an alternative program to the basic sciences called problem-based learning (PBL). This instructional method involves learning in the context of solving a real problem. PBL was initially designed to help medical school students learn basic sciences in a lasting way, and to develop clinical skills simultaneously. So much more than just book learning, this revolutionary method uses actual clinical cases based on actual patients to stimulate inquiry, critical thinking, and knowledge application as it integrates biological, behavioral, and social sciences. This case-based approach means that the student does not have to wait until the final 2 years of medical school to gain an understanding of how to treat actual patients. Through study of clinical cases, this highly effective learning process helps students to acquire a deeper understanding of the principles of medicine and, more important, the skills necessary for lifelong learning.

I believe the breadth of knowledge and recall I gained with PBL was far superior to traditional methods. My retention of what I was studying in anatomy, physiology, pathology, and pharmacology was astonishing. This method greatly accelerated my pace of learning, enabling me to graduate in 3 years instead of the traditional 4. I passed all my exams with flying colors. Finishing med school a year early was important to me. With a family to support in Connecticut, tuition and living expenses were a financial burden.

CHOOSING DIRECTION

My time working with children at the Muscular Dystrophy Association motivated me to apply for a pediatrics residency. Having grown up in Connecticut, I was pleased to be accepted to the pediatric residency at Yale University in New Haven. Dr. Sidney Hurwitz, associate clinical professor of pediatrics and dermatology at Yale School of Medicine, became a close friend and mentor. He had been a pediatrician for a decade before he returned to a residency in dermatology. He encouraged me to consider a dermatology residency as well. He advised that I could treat both children and adults as well as perform surgery with those credentials.

And so my career began. I spent decades in private practice, was an assistant professor at Yale, and served as chief of dermatology at the Connecticut State Veterans Hospital. I had many other positions and appointments as a board-certified dermatologist. My studies and research in nutrition earned me the highly sought-after title of master of the American College of Nutrition. During these years, my focus became finely tuned. The discoveries I first made in medical school, especially in my histopathology classes, became increasingly relevant and significant. These observations became the cornerstone of my clinical practice. The discoveries not only shaped my medical practice but also gave me direction for ongoing research.

EARLY OBSERVATION OF THE INFLAMMATION-AGING CONNECTION

To learn more about the hundreds of diseases covered in our textbooks, we had to look at microscopic studies of normal and diseased tissue. This is called histopathology. The process was examining the patient (a clinical exam) and then taking a biopsy if necessary and examining it under the microscope. This would result in the clinical and microscopic correlation needed to determine the correct diagnosis.

When I observed various inflammatory diseases, such as cancers, invariably there was microscopic inflammation at the cellular level. I questioned my professors, wondering if the inflammation could be triggering or promoting cancer and many other diseases. My questions were dismissed with the explanation that the immune system was reacting to the presence of the disease and not acting as the cause. I asked if there could be more to it than that, because the inflammation was present even when the cancer was not full-blown. I had observed inflammation with precancers under the microscope. I asked if an inflammatory response could be triggering or promoting cancer or the many other diseases I was observing. My questions again were dismissed out of hand.

Medical students are quick to learn that discretion is the better part of valor, and that topics like this are not open for debate. Nor does a medical student's opinion have much weight. But I just could not accept that answer. It was not just cancer and precancer that showed inflammation under the microscope. I observed biopsies of all organ systems, including the liver, heart, brain, and arteries; many showed signs of inflammation microscopically. Inflammation was seen in arteries of patients with atherosclerosis and heart disease. There was also inflammation visible under the microscope when looking at postmortem (autopsy) brain tissue from patients with cognitive decline and Alzheimer's.

During my dermatology residency, once again we looked at skin diseases and clinical signs of aging under the microscope. Inflammation was present. Yet skin without clinical signs of aging or disease showed no inflammation. This discovery so intrigued me that I began to search for ways to put my emerging theory to the test. That was the beginning of my inflammation-aging-disease theory.

Under the microscope, the inflammatory cells of the immune system have an unmistakable appearance. In order to make these cells visible we stain the slide with a blue dye. The inflammation shows as dark blue dots, like confetti—although the presence of inflammation is nothing to celebrate.

This "confetti" also appears when we look at aging skin. I was puzzled about why this was occurring. I wondered if inflammation could be causing these changes. I began to consider wrinkles and other signs of aging skin as a disease, because inflammation was present when damage to skin tissue resulted in wrinkles.

Whenever I looked with a microscope at everything from arthritis to heart disease, inflammation was always a component. Every disease I studied had a common theme; whether it was cancer or aging, inflammation was present. This inflammation was subclinical, invisible to the naked eye, but it goes on day after day, eventually causing great damage to all organ systems.

I was convinced that the inflammation I was finding was not a secondary response, as my professors had suggested. I believed inflammation to be the key to disease of every type. This led me to develop an inflammation-aging-disease theory that has been the basis my research for decades.

I began to search for safe, effective anti-inflammatories to stop, treat, and reverse the symptoms without doing harm. My background in nutrition led me to consider antioxidants as a possible therapeutic approach. All antioxidants are anti-inflammatories, but not all anti-inflammatories are antioxidants, an example of which is ibuprofen.

In dermatology, signs of aging and disease are very visible. I have made it my life's work to intervene. My goal has been to halt inflammation, reversing its negative effects internally and externally. That goal sparked my revolutionary course of study, which influenced and directed my research, resulting in more than 200 US patents, multiple bestsellers and public television specials, and a life purpose and mission that drives me to this day.

THE BRAIN-BEAUTY CONNECTION: FINDING THE MISSING LINK

During my psychiatry rotation in medical school, I observed changes in the skin of patients who were on psychotropic medications. This type of medication affects how the brain works, causing changes in mood, awareness, thoughts, feelings, or behavior. I was simultaneously taking courses in histopathology, in which I examined tissue under a microscope. I could see clearly that the structure of skin tissue was very similar to that of brain tissue. I remembered my embryology course teaching that the skin and nervous system are derived from a single sheet of cells called ectoderm. Put simply, in an embryonic state, layers of cells that eventually develop into skin are also responsible for making brain cells. This means that the skin and brain are very closely connected.

I refer to this as the brain-beauty connection. Much more than a protective barrier, the skin has receptor sites for many types of messengers. Not only can the skin transmit messages throughout the body, but it can also receive messages by way of neurotransmitters, neuropeptides, hormones, and nerve impulses. This information-superhighway communication system opens doors to a greater understanding of the mind-body connection and its role in physical and mental health.

The connection is relevant when we look at diseases of the skin as well as mental diseases and disorders. By stimulating the skin, you can change the chemistry of your brain. Conversely, anxiety attacks, depression, and other mental and psychological stressors will affect the appearance of your skin. Acne, rosacea, psoriasis, eczema or atopic dermatitis, and hair loss are just a few of the skin disorders that have been associated with increased rates of depression, anxiety, and reduced energy. Some of the skin conditions frequently linked to mental health and stress include acne, psoriasis, and eczema.

Historically, many skin diseases are difficult to treat because many have an unknown etiology, or origin. We know that these diseases have a significant inflammatory component. Any acne sufferer will tell you that new lesions always appear before an important event—and that is no coincidence. This expands the truth of the aphorism "you are what you eat" to "you are what you think and feel."

These observations put my imagination into overdrive. I began to consider whether classic therapeutic interventions for brain health would be applicable in treating the skin, because many of these medications possessed antioxidant and/or anti-inflammatory properties.

I looked into DMAE, a psychoactive molecule available by prescription for treating attention deficit disorder. DMAE later became widely available in health food stores for cognitive enhancement. It has become known as a mind health compound that protects brain function, improves memory, and enhances skin health, which should come as no surprise given the brain-beauty connection.

Studies have shown that DMAE enhances synthesis of acetylcholine. This allows the brain to optimize production of acetylcholine, which is essential for learning and memory. When DMAE increases acetylcholine production, muscle tone improves. Good muscle tone is evident when we are young. We can maintain this appearance by using DMAE either orally or topically.

DMAE can protect neurons and other cells from the harmful effects of certain types of oxidation by stabilizing the cell plasma membrane, which acts as an antioxidant. In addition, DMAE sustains metabolic processes in the body by means of a process known as methyl donation. My ideas about the brain-beauty connection led me to work and formulate with DMAE.

DMAE became a cornerstone ingredient in a line of anti-aging skin treatments I developed decades ago, all thanks to that aha! moment during my residency, when I realized that what is therapeutic for the brain can be equally therapeutic and healing for the skin. DMAE is instrumental in increasing the production of acetylcholine, the Beauty Molecule, the heart and soul of this book.

UNDERSTANDING AGING

Most people think that skin aging is caused by chronological age. We assume that the older we are in years, the more wrinkled we will be. But the truth is not that simple. Many other lifestyle factors contribute to, or accelerate, skin aging and can make us look years older than our chronological age. At the same time, young people with acne, who may not show any signs of chronological aging, can have all the signs of an inflammatory response.

UNDERSTANDING HOW WE AGE

Lifestyle factors that fuel chronic inflammation, age your skin, and promote disease include:

- Diet high in sugar and simple carbohydrates
- Environmental stressors
- Weakened immune system
- Excess exposure to sun and other sources of ultraviolet light
- Hormonal changes
- Stress
- Smoking

Inflammation exists in a broad spectrum ranging from low to high. On the low side, it occurs on a cellular level and can be discerned only microscopically, or submicroscopically on a molecular level. Even low-level inflammation can be highly damaging. Chronic, subclinical inflammation is behind skin problems from acne to enlarged pores, from wrinkles and sagging to loss of tone and radiance. Chronic inflammation also compromises the function of all other organ systems. On the high side of the spectrum, the inflammation is visibly evident—for example, the redness and swelling of a wound or sunburn.

EXTERNAL SIGNS OF CHRONIC INFLAMMATION

Skin problems are telltale signs of internal inflammation. Unlike the internal organs, the deterioration of skin cells is highly visible. We are all familiar with that deterioration.

My life's work has been to prevent and correct the universal signs of aging that result from the passage of time, environmental exposure, genetics, epigenetics, and lifestyle.

Chronic inflammation can affect your skin in many ways, manifesting as:

- Loss of elasticity
- Thinner, more translucent skin
- Wrinkles
- Dry, rough, leathery skin
- Broken capillaries on the face
- Freckles
- Pigmented spots on the face, on the back of the hands, and on the arms, chest, and upper back
- Puffiness
- Lack of radiance
- Sagging
- Deep lines
- Loss of firmness
- Enlarged pores

Beautiful, glowing skin is the most visible sign of good health.

Chronic inflammation can age your skin and make you look older. If you do not like what you see in the mirror, you can do something about it. In *The Beauty Molecule*, I give you several strategies for avoiding or combating these undesirable, aging effects.

THE BIRTH OF A WRINKLE

Inflammation does its damage by triggering free radicals, which accelerate aging by damaging cells. Free radicals are molecules that have lost an electron in interactions with other molecules. As a result, these molecules are extremely unstable or reactive. Driven to become whole, free radicals steal

ET

ntal clar-
ding to an
on. When
nefits, in-

diseases
nd heart

mmatory

e in blood
void foods
release of

s, creating more free radicals and damag-
ss.

high level of free radicals, the condition is
stress leads to the production of chemicals
the cell. This stressed state also activates
ase that break down proteins like collagen
skin and make it supple. When those pro-
es, becoming wrinkled, dry, and leathery.
s, microscarring occurs—and there we have

nly a nanosecond and does very little direct
n their very brief lives, free radicals initiate
h can continue for hours or even days. The
scade results in most of the cellular damage
d diseases.

age to the mitochondria, the part of the cell
tion of cellular rejuvenation. A young cell is
gy production. Slow down that production,
ss.

llular metabolism—the chemical and phys-
our body builds and maintains itself, and by
l nutrients to produce energy.

interest in nutrition encouraged me to con-
a major cause of inflammation. Foods and
in our mental and physical health and well-
food choice is the common denominator of so
ases, ranging from wrinkled skin to obesity to
se to depression, from aging to acne.

THE BENEFITS OF AN ANTI-INFLAMMATORY DI

Controlling inflammation is the key to health, longevity, me
ity, and well-being, and to radiant, youthful skin. Eating accor
anti-inflammatory diet is the best way to conquer inflammat
you follow an anti-inflammatory diet, you will enjoy many be
cluding:

- Losing weight and maintaining a healthy weight for life
- Maintaining muscle mass
- Beautifying your skin
- Elevating your mood
- Improving your brain function
- Increasing your energy
- Improving your athletic ability
- Protecting yourself from a wide range of degenerative
  associated with aging, like Alzheimer's disease, arthritis,
  disease
- Living life to the fullest

This list should be enough to motivate you to give the anti-infla
diet a try.

The anti-inflammatory diet is designed to prevent a rapid ri
sugar. When you are eating to fight inflammation, you must a
that provoke a glycemic response in your body and a subsequen
insulin, which in turn triggers an inflammatory response.

FOODS THAT FUEL INFLAMMATION

Foods are converted to sugar at varying rates. Those that are rapidly converted to sugar, including sugary and starchy foods, beverages, and processed foods, are pro-inflammatory. Foods that are pro-inflammatory include:

- Candy
- All processed foods
- Breads, pastry, croissants, cookies, pies, and other baked goods
- Pasta
- Snack foods like potato and corn chips, pretzels, and rice cakes
- Sugary sodas, fruit juice, and sports drinks
- Alcoholic beverages

The inflammatory response caused by these foods results in the acceleration of the aging process of all organ systems in your body, increasing the risk of degenerative disease and wrinkled, sagging skin.

Pro-inflammatory foods might form a large portion of your diet and serve as comfort food. At this point, the thought of doing without foods that have become mainstays may seem a big sacrifice. I assure you that the benefits of eating an anti-inflammatory diet will outweigh any sacrifice you think you are making.

As a dermatologist, I am naturally most excited about the results visible in the skin, but there are a great many benefits to eating this way. The collateral benefits affect all organ systems, enhancing and maintaining cognitive function, restoring energy, decreasing cardiovascular diseases, regulating body fat, and reducing the risk of metabolic diseases such as diabetes.

AXULIN—A GENUINE SCIENTIFIC
BREAKTHROUGH

While attending a recent conference in Miami, I ran into an old friend and colleague, Dr. Mehmet Oz. We had not seen each other in a number of years. I was delighted to accept an invitation to lunch with him and his wife, Lisa. We were joined by another guest, Dr. Gerard Housey. It came as no surprise that Mehmet would have such an exciting and accomplished friend and colleague.

I learned that Dr. Housey holds a doctorate in human genetics as well as being a licensed physician. He has conducted cancer research at the National Cancer Institute of the National Institutes of Health. A committed researcher and inventor, Dr. Housey is the president and CEO of Housey Pharmaceutical Research Laboratories, where he directs the company's research and development programs. One of his most important inventions is a target-specific cell-based assay system, a technology currently in widespread use in the pharmaceutical industry.

During lunch, Dr. Housey discussed his recent invention, Axulin, a nonprescription therapeutic supplement he developed as a nutritional support for diabetes, metabolic syndrome, polycystic ovarian syndrome, and prediabetes. Plant-based Axulin is formulated to maintain healthy blood sugar levels and metabolize carbohydrates and fats. I was excited to learn that Axulin mimics the effects of the anti-inflammatory diet. Dr. Housey explained that Axulin works on the insulin receptor IRS2. He told us that laboratory and clinical studies have shown that Axulin provides support for the body's glucose-regulating process by targeting the same pathway that insulin uses to control blood sugar.

I knew that insulin signaling is controlled mainly by that IRS2 protein, which is activated when insulin binds to an insulin receptor on a cell's surface. This activation stimulates glucose uptake from the blood, reducing blood sugar levels, which is a good thing. An increase in blood sugar produces an insulin response that results in increased inflammation on a cellular level.

My anti-inflammatory diet is designed to give us the complete spectrum of nutrients and, at the same time, carefully control insulin and blood sugar. In all of my books, I have emphasized the importance of controlling our blood sugar and insulin levels as a key to maintaining our beauty and health. A tablet that will ensure blood sugar control is truly a game changer!

I was excited to realize that this supplement was a genuine "magic bullet," one that I had been in search of for years. Axulin changes the way we metabolize blood sugar while maintaining tight control of insulin, which could prevent type 1 and type 2 diabetes. From my perspective, the ability to control insulin is a significant anti-aging strategy.

As you know, a well-controlled diet can make a big difference in the total burden of inflammation in the body, reducing our risk of all diseases, including aging. I did not hesitate to say to Dr. Housey, Dr. Oz, and Lisa that I believed the invention of Axulin was worthy of the Nobel Prize. Chronic, subclinical inflammation ultimately results in a host of progressive diseases. Dr. Housey's vegetable-based, nontoxic, inexpensive tablet may well be the ultimate anti-aging and anti-inflammatory strategy—with the power to change our lives in a positive way.

I predict that Axulin will become an indispensable adjunct for a variety of inflammatory issues in the body. In addition, I believe that Axulin will make a powerful contribution in the efforts of science to prevent cognitive decline as we age. I am grateful to Mehmet Oz and Lisa for their invaluable introduction to Dr. Gerald Housey and for giving me the opportunity to share this breakthrough with you. To learn more about this genuine scientific gift to us all, visit Axulin.com.

The anti-inflammatory diet is such an important anti-aging strategy that I am devoting the following chapter to the details of eating to combat inflammation. An anti-inflammatory diet is a powerful tool for supporting the Beauty Molecule to protect the mitochondria and repair damaged cells.

A review of the basics of this life-changing way of eating, which is the at the core of my program, is in order.

3

THE NUTRITIONAL FACELIFT
AND SO MUCH MORE

THE BEST STRATEGY FOR STAYING healthy and keeping your skin youthful and radiant is to follow an anti-inflammatory diet designed to control blood sugar and insulin levels and to prevent the production of free radicals. One of the secrets of the success of the dietary recommendations I first introduced in *The Wrinkle Cure* is the diet's ability to control the amount of insulin and blood sugar produced from the foods we eat. This is critical because controlling blood sugar and insulin is how to control systemic inflammation.

. . . .

FUNDAMENTALS OF THE ANTI-INFLAMMATORY DIET

The best way to stay at peak health and radiant beauty is to eat in a way that quiets systemic inflammation. The general range of foods that should be the staples of your diet include:

- High-quality protein, like that found in fish, shellfish, poultry, and tofu
- Low-glycemic carbohydrates in moderation, including colorful fresh fruits, vegetables, whole grains, and legumes. The cruciferous

vegetables like cabbage, broccoli, and cauliflower are strong anti-inflammatories.
- Healthful fats like those from cold-water fish—especially wild Alaskan salmon, halibut, sardines, herring, and anchovies—and in nuts, seeds, and olive oil
- Two 8-ounce cans of hydrogen water (the importance of which is covered in chapter 6) a day
- 6 to 8 glasses of pure spring water a day
- Antioxidant-rich beverages such as green tea, as well as white and black tea

These foods and beverages are natural anti-inflammatories. Ideally, they will be the cornerstone of your diet. Once you start eating this way, you will experience positive changes in your appearance, energy, and mood. You will be on the right path to increased health span and lasting beauty.

It may now seem hard to believe that the statements I made in *The Wrinkle Cure* were highly controversial at the time, and not generally accepted by the academic community. The popular diet then was the no-fat/low-fat fad, which has since been proven to be harmful and unhealthful. That diet fad was counterintuitive to everything I knew to be true. We need the right kind of fats for healthy brain function, for our immune system, and for burning fat.

THE SKIN AS A BAROMETER OF HEALTH

In my roles as a dermatologist and nutritionist, I observed over many years that the skin gave me a clear picture of whether my patients were eating correctly and leading a healthful lifestyle. I noticed that when I placed patients on the anti-inflammatory diet for just 3 days, there was an obvious difference in the quality of their skin. The skin showed increased radiance, tightening of pores, and increased overall tone. I know that it is difficult to believe that just 3 days can make a visible difference in the skin, but you must understand that the skin is the ideal barometer to reflect the health of the internal organs.

When we decrease inflammation in our bodies, not only does our skin look much better, but also our mind is clear, because all our organ systems function more efficiently. The mitochondria are improving our energy levels. Because inflammation is the final common pathway of all disease processes, including aging, it is encouraging to realize how much control we have in its prevention or progression. We can lead an anti-inflammatory lifestyle that will enable us to live life to the fullest. This allows us, regardless of our chronological age, to manifest true beauty, which is nothing more than radiant health.

THE 3-DAY FACELIFT

Even seasoned and difficult-to-impress media journalists, like Oprah Winfrey and Diane Sawyer, could not believe their eyes when they witnessed the effects of the anti-inflammatory diet after just 3 days.

The test subjects on the *Oprah Winfrey Show*, chosen by the show's producers, all were transformed. Their luminous skin made them look younger and feel more energetic than they had been a scant 72 hours earlier. Three women from the audience shared their before and after photos. The women appeared in person to attest to the miracle of the anti-inflammatory diet. I am not exaggerating when I say there was an audible gasp from the audience as the results were revealed.

The same dramatic transformations were seen on *Good Morning America*. The producers of that show named the experiment "Is There a Face Lift in Your Fridge?" Before my appearance on the "reveal" segment, Diane Sawyer told me that she felt my claims were overstated and that she planned to challenge me. Her doubt did not shake my confidence. I knew that as long as the candidates had not cheated, the diet would have its effect. When we approached the subjects, who were about fifty yards from us, Diane stopped in her tracks. In a tone of disbelief, she exclaimed, "I can see a difference from here!"

Seeing a visible difference in your looks in just 3 days may seem too good to be true, but if you eat the wrinkle-free way for even a short period of time, you will experience dramatic changes not only in how you look but also in how you feel. My recommendations for what to eat for 3 days are very specific. The focus on salmon; salads with extra-virgin olive oil, fresh, dark leafy greens, and berries; and plenty of spring water are the core of the 3-day program.

After the television trials aired, there was a run on salmon and blueberries in stores across the country. And *The Wrinkle Cure* hit the #1 spot on the *New York Times* bestseller list the following Sunday.

The 3-day nutritional facelift is the perfect way to jump-start a longer commitment to healthful eating. This will allow you to see visible results in your skin right away. Or you can use this diet as a stand-alone quick fix—especially if you have an important event, party, reunion, job interview, or big date, and want to look your best. Not only will you see rapid changes in your skin, but you will also notice a boost in your mood and energy levels.

THE 3-DAY NUTRITIONAL FACELIFT

The 3-day facelift helps to eliminate puffiness, increase contours, and firm the jawline. The diet acts as a natural diuretic, reducing the puffiness seen on the faces of the majority of people who consume the average American diet.

You must eat salmon at least twice a day for the ideal effect. This will change your skin, making it firmer and more lustrous. Wild salmon is far superior to farm-raised salmon, but farm-raised salmon will still give you benefits. In many ways, salmon is the perfect food because it provides high-quality, easily absorbed protein. Protein supplies the amino acids, such as taurine, necessary to repair the body on a cellular level. Recent research has shown that high levels of taurine can increase lifespan up to 20 percent. A carbohydrate-heavy and protein-light diet leads to the loss of contours in the face—the sought-after chiseled look of a well-defined jawline, cheekbones, and eyes.

Salmon is also an excellent source of the essential fatty acids EPA and DHA, which are vital for brain function; for mood health; for the metabolism of fats, which help to control excess body fat; and for the beauty of your skin.

It is no secret that I am a huge fan of wild salmon. Many people refer to me as the "salmon and blueberry doctor." Wild salmon and other cold-water fish are great sources of protein, necessary to maintain and repair the body on a cellular level The lack of protein is first visible in the face, especially as we age, but the same is true for young people.

On the days you do not have adequate protein, your rate of aging accelerates.

Drinking two 8-ounce cans of hydrogen water in the morning is optional. I explain the outstanding benefits of this all-purpose health booster, hydrogen water, in chapter 6, and encourage you to add it to your diet.

Some guidelines to follow for optimal results include:

- No substitutions for any foods listed
- Drink at least 6 glasses of pure water a day
- Always eat protein first, as it helps slow down carbohydrate absorption, which results in control of insulin and glucose levels. I will be repeating this statement many times. The key to the anti-inflammatory diet is to carefully control blood sugar and insulin. This is because a spike in glucose levels causes an insulin response, resulting in inflammation on a cellular level that can last for up to 3 days.

THE 3-DAY NUTRITIONAL DIET

BREAKFAST

2-egg omelet, or 4 to 6 ounces grilled, baked, or poached salmon
(I do not recommend smoked salmon on the 3-day diet because of the
high salt content. Otherwise, smoked salmon is fine.)

2-inch slice cantaloupe or ⅓ cup fresh berries

6 to 8 ounces spring water (feel free to squeeze fresh lemon into the
water if desired)

No juice, coffee, or toast

If you normally have coffee to start your day, drink black or green tea to
prevent caffeine withdrawal.

LUNCH

4 to 6 ounces grilled, baked, or poached poultry

2 cups green salad, made with romaine lettuce and other dark, leafy
greens such as spinach, arugula, and kale. Top with 3 tablespoons
cooked chickpeas. (Canned chickpeas are fine as long as you drain
them.)

Extra-virgin olive oil dressing, with fresh-squeezed lemon to taste

1 apple, or 1 pear, or 2-inch slice cantaloupe, or ⅓ cup berries

6 to 8 ounces spring water

DINNER

4 to 6 ounces freshly cooked—grilled, broiled, or poached—salmon on
1 cup of warmed lentils

Green salad (as described above)

½ cup steamed vegetables, especially asparagus, broccoli, and spinach
(avoid root vegetables like potatoes, carrots, beets, and parsnips)

2-inch slice cantaloupe

6 to 8 ounces spring water

If you follow this diet for 3 days to the letter, be ready for a great improvement in how you look and feel.

. . . .

Of course, science has advanced in the 22 years since *The Wrinkle Cure* was published. We now have a greater understanding of the mechanisms that control inflammation. Rather than traversing old ground, *The Beauty Molecule* covers new facts about the role of healing and rejuvenating foods. We now have scientific data at the molecular level that illustrates why the salmon, salads, berries, green tea, and extra-virgin olive oil in the 3-day diet, along with all anti-inflammatory foods, are so successful in slowing aging and preventing disease. We explore the specific relationship to the Beauty Molecule of each of these foods. Because the role of inflammation in aging and disease is now widely accepted, there is much current and ongoing research that gives us a fresh view of what happens within the body when inflammation is unchecked.

For the balance of this chapter, I want to go deeper to take a close look at how an anti-inflammatory works to fight inflammation. We will take a look at other anti-inflammatory foods that protect and restore the mitochondria, stimulate the parasympathetic nervous system, and eliminate old and damaged cells.

. . . .

A VICAR'S TALE

Father James, an ordained priest in the Church of England, first came to see me as a patient when he was 38 years old. He was visiting relatives in the US who were concerned about his health. At the time of our first appointment, Father James had been serving as a missionary in developing countries for nearly 10 years.

His main complaint concerned skin rashes that had intermittently plagued him during the past several years. Father James was more accustomed to providing spiritual healing than receiving physical healing, a reason for his long delay in seeking treatment. Upon the urging of his concerned family members, he made an appointment to see me. And that was the start of a twenty-plus-years doctor-patient relationship.

The physical examination showed simple, inflamed areas of the skin, which I diagnosed as contact dermatitis. The fact that the vicar demonstrated all the signs of protein deficiency did not escape my attention. When we discussed his work in developing countries, his diet as a missionary was far from adequate, as I suspected. When he had returned to Europe, he contracted the SARS virus, which left him with inflammation around his heart.

I could see that this clergyman was extremely dedicated to his work—to the point of neglecting his own health as he helped others. I wanted to do more than simply treat his skin eruptions. I told him of my concern about his diet and how his physical exam revealed signs of a protein deficiency. I went on to explain that we need adequate protein on a daily basis in order for cells to repair themselves, and that ongoing lack of protein accelerates aging. I told him I was acutely aware of this because lack of adequate protein is first visible in the face. Sagging and loss of firmness and youthful contours are signs of protein deprivation, aging the face even more than pronounced wrinkles. But all organ systems are negatively affected by lack of protein. Unfortunately, his ongoing protein deficiency was risky for his SARS-damaged heart.

Protein, the building block of life, cannot be stored in the body. It needs to be eaten every day at each meal. Fish, shellfish, poultry, grass-fed and pasture-raised meats, eggs, and dairy products are excellent sources of high-quality protein. Our muscles, organs, bones, cartilage, skin, and the antibodies that protect us from disease are all made of protein. Even the enzymes that facilitate essential chemical reactions in the body—from digestion to building cells—are made of protein. If our cells do not have complete availability of all the essential amino acids, cellular repair will slow down and be incomplete.

Without adequate protein, our bodies enter into an accelerated aging mode. Although not even 40, Father James had lost muscle mass and his hair was thinning. He seemed tired, frail, and weak. His skin showed signs of losing elasticity. Father James's face and body looked as if they belonged to a significantly older man. All these signs pointed to inadequate protein.

We spent some time talking about improvements he needed to make to his diet, and nutritional supplements that would help to rebuild the damage caused by the past decade of inadequate nutrition and his work in a physically and mentally stressful environment. I explained to Father James that if he did not follow my advice, which was supported by the cardiologist with whom I consulted, the long-term prognosis was not good.

He took my advice to heart. Upon returning to the UK, he accepted a position as a vicar with a small parish church 30 minutes west of London, rather than continuing his far-flung missionary work. When he returned to the US to visit his relatives, Father James made an appointment for a follow-up visit. I was delighted to see that his health and overall appearance were significantly improved. He looked robust and 10 years younger. Having seen the cardiologist, he was happy to report that the pericarditis, the SARS-related inflammation around the heart, was quite stable.

TRUE COLORS

Among the powerful benefits you gain from a diet full of brightly colored fruits and vegetables are their antioxidant properties. An antioxidant inhibits oxidation, a chemical reaction that can produce free radicals.

The best-known antioxidants are carotenoids and polyphenols. Examples of each include:

CAROTENOIDS	POLYPHENOLS
Beta-carotene	Anthocyanidans
Lycopene	Catechins
Lutein	Flavonoids
Zeaxanthin	Tannins
Astaxanthin	Hydroxytyrosol

Carotenoids are fat-soluble pigments that give red/yellow/orange color to fruits, vegetables, egg yolks, salmon, steelhead trout, shellfish, and the feathers of birds, notably brilliant pink flamingos. Fish and fowl alike get their red/yellow/orange hues from eating large quantities of carotenoid-rich aquatic plants like algae and plankton.

Dark, leafy greens like spinach, kale, chard, and collards also are rich in carotenoids, but their red/yellow/orange colors are masked by green-hued chlorophyll, which is a more dominant pigment.

Carotenoids play a significant role in cellular growth and repair. Their fat solubility allows them to enter the cell plasma membrane and the mitochondria, which is very important for protecting our immune systems. Immune cells are particularly sensitive to oxidative stress. The importance of the ability of the carotenoids to penetrate the cell cannot be overemphasized, now that we know that damage to the mitochondria is where aging begins.

The carotenoid family of antioxidants offers special and targeted properties for cellular rejuvenation. These antioxidants have an important role in cellular growth and repair. Fruits and vegetables are usually considered the best source of carotenoids, but astaxanthin, a carotenoid found in fish and fowl, is what gives wild salmon its deep red or bright pink hue. Astaxanthin helps to make salmon a superfood that can single-handedly deliver optimal health to the entire body, including the skin—and that means youthful, glowing skin.

Carotenoids in general, and astaxanthin specifically, neutralize free radicals. Astaxanthin has the ability to protect the cell membrane from free radicals, specifically the reactive oxygen species or ROS, including the hydroxyl radical, the most damaging of all.

Often referred to as the king of carotenoids, astaxanthin defends against the most damaging oxidative insults to our bodies. Astaxanthin provides powerful protection to the mitochondria as well as to the lipid bilayer that surrounds the cells and the organelles within, such as the nucleus. Unique to astaxanthin, this dual protection is one reason this antioxidant plays such an important role in protecting the cells from inflammation. Astaxanthin can penetrate all portions of the cell, which enables it to protect organs and systems throughout the body. This broad-based protection is the foundation for its anti-aging properties.

Recent studies have confirmed that astaxanthin acts powerfully in the brain, because it is able to cross the blood-brain barrier. Astaxanthin has been found to be a promising therapeutic anti-inflammatory agent for many neurological disorders, including cerebral ischemia, Parkinson's disease, Alzheimer's disease, autism, and neuropathic pain.

THE HEALING EFFECT OF CRUCIFEROUS VEGETABLES

You most likely know to make sure you eat plenty of cruciferous vegetables, like broccoli, cabbage, cauliflower, brussels sprouts, bok choy, watercress, collard greens, and arugula. The phytochemical that gives cruciferous vegetables their power is indole-3-carbinol, also called I3C. The chemical is converted in the stomach to antioxidants and powerful stimulators of natural detoxifying enzymes. Indole-3-carbinol boosts DNA repair in cells and may even stop them from becoming cancerous. This is a critical finding because DNA is the material inside the nucleus of cells that carries genetic information. If we are genetically predisposed to cancer, it may prove possible to repair our cells and prevent cancer simply by eating broccoli. Scientists are ardently pursuing this fascinating premise, which is one more reason to eat those cruciferous vegetables.

POLYPHENOLS: CELLULAR BEAUTY SECRETS

Berries, which are rich in polyphenols, are another important component of an anti-inflammatory diet. Some of the most common polyphenols—such as those found in many fruits, vegetables, tea, and cocoa—exhibit substantial antioxidant protection at the cell membrane, where it counts.

Research conducted during the past decade has provided ample evidence that the water-soluble polyphenol antioxidants in some foods and herbs, often grouped under the umbrella term "flavonoids," also provide substantial protection against free radical damage to cell membranes. This is highly significant because reducing the number of free radicals in the cell membrane protects the mitochondria.

The more colorful the food we eat, the higher the polyphenol content. Fruits, especially berries, and vegetables are excellent sources of polyphenols. These polyphenols can normalize blood pressure and reduce excess abdominal fat, which decreases the risk of heart disease. Polyphenols contribute to rapidly increasing visible radiance of the skin.

GREEN TEA

Another staple of Perricone-recommended foods and beverages is green tea, rich in catechin polyphenols including EGCG, which is short for epigallocatechin gallate. EGCG eliminates inflammation-producing free radicals. Polyphenols protect healthy cells from cancer caused by DNA damage, while ushering cancer cells to their death. These polyphenols can help in the healing of skin diseases such as psoriasis, ulcers, rosacea, and wounds—and wrinkles. The benefits of green tea also include improved brain function, fat loss, and lower risk of heart disease.

If you are a coffee drinker, these are good reasons to switch to green tea. You can still indulge in coffee now and then.

Green tea, strawberries, blue- and blackberries, apples, and cocoa are among the antioxidant foods high in catechins, antioxidants that protect the skin from UV damage. The deeper and richer the color, the higher the catechin content.

YES TO NO (NITRIC OXIDE)

The foods and beverages I have been recommending for many years stimulate synthesis of the signaling gas nitric oxide (NO). This is the secret to why the salmon and salads give a dramatic increase in radiance. Nitric oxide, produced by nearly every type of cell in the human body, is one of the most important molecules for blood vessel health. As a vasodilator, NO relaxes the inner muscles of your blood vessels, causing the vessels to widen. Critical to our cardiovascular health, nitric oxide increases blood flow and lowers blood pressure.

Several foods enhance the bioavailability of nitric oxide. But be aware that the use of mouthwash will kill the friendly bacteria that are necessary to convert nitrates to nitrites, which are then converted to nitric oxide. Some of those foods, and their active ingredients, are:

- **Garlic** boosts nitric oxide levels by activating nitric oxide synthase, the enzyme that helps to convert the amino acid L-arginine to nitric oxide
- **Meat, poultry, and seafood** are sources of coenzyme Q10 (CoQ10), a compound that helps preserve nitric oxide in the body
- **Dark chocolate,** thanks to the flavonols found in cocoa, helps to keep nitric oxide at an optimal level
- **Leafy green vegetables** are loaded with nitrates, which are converted to nitric oxide
- **Citrus fruits** are good sources of vitamin C, which increases the bioavailability of nitric oxide and maximizes its absorption in the body
- **Pomegranates** are full of powerful antioxidants that protect

nitric oxide from oxidative damage, increase levels of nitric oxide synthase, and increase the concentration of nitrites in the blood

- **Nuts and seeds** contain arginine, an amino acid involved in the production of nitric oxide
- **Watermelon** is a good source of citrulline, an amino acid that is converted to nitric-oxide-producing arginine
- **Red wine**, in moderation of course, contains potent antioxidants that increase nitric oxide synthase levels, resulting in increased production of nitric oxide

Not only does nitric oxide protect cardiovascular health, but its promotion of better circulation will also give your skin a glow that can be seen across the room.

LIQUID GOLD: EXTRA-VIRGIN OLIVE OIL

An important Perricone-recommended food, extra-virgin olive oil is one of the most powerful anti-inflammatory foods on the list. Extra-virgin olive oil contains a powerful antioxidant called hydroxytyrosol. After a lifetime of research, I have begun to believe that olive oil (along with hydrogen water) bubbled up from the fountain of youth.

The right kinds of fats, like those found in olive oil or salmon, play a tremendous role in how well we age. Many find this hard to believe because fat has been so vilified in our lifetime, but my statement is true. At the same time, not all fats and lipids are as good for you as those found in extra-virgin olive oil and salmon. I do not recommend corn, canola, cottonseed, soy, safflower, sunflower, grapeseed, and rice bran oils, which can be pro-inflammatory. Many fats are toxic—the trans fats found in so many processed foods, for example. Our fat choices are important because both the "good" and "bad" fats rapidly penetrate the cells, either to our great benefit or serious detriment. The good fats exert an anti-inflammatory effect on our cells and will prevent cell breakdown. On the other hand, the bad fats, such as the man-made trans fats, exert an immediate pro-inflammatory response, aging your cells and you along with it.

HIGH-FAT/BAD-FAT DIET AND MITOCHONDRIAL DAMAGE

A diet high in the wrong fats can compromise the mitochondria, which are necessary for all life. When we look at an electron microscope photo of the mitochondria damaged from a high-fat diet in animal models, we can see that the perfectly formed oval organoid shape of the mitochondria lose its vertical lines and begin to have a distorted appearance. This means that the energy-producing portion of the mitochondria has been compromised, which has profound effects on our cells and organ systems. When scientists increased the amount of the Beauty Molecule, acetylcholine, in the compromised animals, they found that the mitochondria were completely repaired in a few months, maintaining perfect shape and function. The scientists did this by administering the medication pyridostigmine, which interferes with acetylcholinesterase, the enzyme that breaks down the Beauty Molecule. Inhibiting acetylcholinesterase results in the need for higher levels of the Beauty Molecule to work efficiently in repairing the mitochondria and reversing the effects of high-fat damage.

PYRIDOSTIGMINE

Pyridostigmine, an acetylcholinesterase inhibitor, is a prescription drug with some remarkable properties. Admittedly, using a prescription drug to illustrate this function is an extreme example. Although I am not advocating its use, I am discussing the drug to show how scientists are searching in our quest to halt and repair the cellular damage that results in aging and disease. When observing the effects of administering pyridostigmine in animal models, researchers have discovered promising results in mitochondrial repair. As you have learned, aging and mitochondrial dysfunction go hand in hand.

The discovery that pyridostigmine can reverse mitochondrial damage in animals by elevating acetylcholine levels clearly indicates that the Beauty Molecule is busy at work repairing the mitochondria. This is the most important point of the book. Throughout *The Beauty Molecule*, especially in part 2, we will illustrate several other strategies for increasing acetylcholine to repair the mitochondria, normalize metabolism, and increase function of all organ systems.

In addition to these important effects, pyridostigmine repairs DNA and assists in cell metabolism. These miraculous functions are activated by increasing the enzyme AMPK, the precursor to the Beauty Molecule.

EXTRA-VIRGIN OLIVE OIL: THE FOUNTAIN OF YOUTH

Current research has shown that a diet rich in anti-inflammatory, antioxidant extra-virgin olive oil affects your health in an abundance of ways. Extra-virgin olive oil has been shown to:

- Increase the skin's ability to maintain moisture
- Correct uneven color when used in topical form
- Increase skin radiance
- Decrease LDL or "bad" cholesterol
- Prevent oxidation of LDL cholesterol by free radicals
- Increase HDL or "good" cholesterol
- Maintain normal blood HDL cholesterol concentrations
- Aid intestinal absorption
- Lower the probability of gallstones
- Lower blood pressure
- Decrease gastric acid secretion in ulcers
- Stimulate pancreas secretion

- Prevent osteoporosis
- Lower glucose levels in diabetics
- Reduce risk of prostate cancer
- Reduce risk of breast cancer
- Be neuroprotective
- Protect the cardiovascular system
- Prevent atherosclerosis
- Regulate glutathione concentration
- Provide antioxidant enzymes to adipose tissue

This impressive list of benefits should convince you that extra-virgin olive oil is liquid gold, and should be your oil of choice.

I must advise you to be diligent about the freshness of oils. Rancid or oxidized fats are extremely toxic and carcinogenic. Your sense of smell is the best way to check freshness. Once open, extra-virgin olive oil lasts between 18 and 24 months. The oil starts to degrade as soon as you open the bottle. For maximum benefits, try to use your extra-virgin olive oil within 6 months. Be sure to store the oil in a cool, dark place. Avoid direct sunlight because heat will turn the oil rancid.

. . . .

THE ACTIVE INGREDIENT IN EVOO

Hydroxytyrosol is one of the most powerful polyphenols. This rare and protective antioxidant is found only in extra-virgin olive oil. Hydroxytyrosol is a by-product obtained from manufacturing olive oil, a compound drawn from the fruit of the olive tree and its leaves. Studies have shown that this compound has 10 times more antioxidant activity than green tea and 2 times more than CoQ10. The molecular structure of hydroxytyrosol enables it to work as an antioxidant, anti-inflammatory, and anti-carcinogen, and as a protector of skin and eyes.

Easily integrated into the body, hydroxytyrosol has a bioavailability of 99 percent. Both water and fat soluble, this powerful antioxidant can more easily penetrate the cellular membrane. The structural and molecular features of hydroxytyrosol ensure that its consumption provides many beneficial effects.

During physical exercise, hydroxytyrosol helps to increase the production of glutathione, the body's master antioxidant, and to reduce the production of lactic acid and the consequent muscular atrophy.

Hydroxytyrosol slows the aging process in the skin by stabilizing the cell plasma membrane. Because it prevents the oxidation of keratin protein, hydroxytyrosol also makes hair soft, shiny, and lustrous, while it prevents nails from peeling and breaking.

In another example of the brain-beauty connection, hydroxytyrosol is protective against the neurodegenerative damage and cognitive decline associated with age or diseases like Alzheimer's or Parkinson's. Hydroxytyrosol protects brain cells from lipid oxidation because it can cross the blood-brain barrier.

HYDROXYTYROSOL ACTIVATES ANTI-AGING GENES

An important function of hydroxytyrosol is to activate anti-aging genes known as sirtuins. Humans have 7 sirtuins, a protein involved in regulating cellular processes, including the aging and death of cells and also their resistance to stress. Proteins belonging to the sirtuin family are one of the most promising strategies for anti-aging.

With enzymatic activity, sirtuins drive reactions forward. When sirtuins were first studied, the focus was on sirtuin 1 (SIRT1), which was believed to have the greatest effect on health and lifespan. The early researchers of SIRT1 believed that resveratrol upregulated SIRT1. Resveratrol is a polyphenol found in red grapes, dark chocolate, and blueberries. SIRT1 activity was eventually found to be not that important, and the early resveratrol studies were probably erroneous.

We now know that sirtuin 6 (SIRT6) has much more effect on lifespan and health span. Our focus is now on SIRT6 and its regulatory functions in aging, cancer, and, especially, immunity. Like SIRT1, SIRT6 resides in the nucleus of the cell.

SIRT6 activity is dependent upon a substance called NAD (nicotinamide adenine dinucleotide), which I will expand upon later. All 7 sirtuins are dependent upon NAD.

Owing to its role in regulating the function of the immune system, SIRT6 can be considered a potential therapeutic target for the treatment of diseases. Studies are showing that SIRT6 is a longevity protein that can inhibit the aging of cells, tissues, organs, and the body by promoting DNA damage repair, maintaining normal chromosome structure, regulating energy metabolism, and reducing inflammatory response. SIRT6 is interesting for its role in preventing inflammatory and metabolic diseases, as well as in cancer.

SIRT6 acts to inhibit the activity of senescent cells, which are cells that eventually stop multiplying but do not die off when they should. Instead, the damaged cells continue to release chemicals that can trigger inflammation in a process known as senescence-associated secretory phenotype (SASP).

Most of the sirtuin 6 studies were done in animal models, but there is good evidence that SIRT6 has a positive effect on our metabolism. It has been shown to increase health span in most of the animal studies. By activating SIRT6 with dietary restriction, drinking hydrogen water, and choosing foods rich in polyphenolic compounds, we can trigger protective activity of sirtuin 6 to normalize metabolism.

Another function of SIRT6 is to prevent frailty, which is a very important risk factor for death. As we age, we become frailer and have more inflammation in our bodies, especially muscle tissue, which leads to a condition of muscle loss known as sarcopenia. This is one of the reasons exercise is an important strategy for longevity. If you can reduce the incidence of fragility and maintain muscle mass and bone density, you will enjoy an increase in health span and, most likely, in lifespan. In the mouse model of aging, SIRT6 elevated lifespan by 27 percent.

Sirtuins appear to play a role during cell response to a variety of stresses, such as oxidative or genotoxic stress. You have read about oxidative stress several times in these pages. Similarly, highly damaging genotoxic stress occurs when chemical agents damage the genetic information within a cell, causing mutations that may lead to cancer. We can add to sirtuin 6's many attributes the important function of regulating DNA repair and maintenance.

In addition, SIRT6 has effects on epigenetics. Epigenetic changes are modifications to DNA that regulate whether genes are turned on or off. These changes either activate or block the activation of a particular gene. As we age, some of the on and off switches do not function perfectly. We end up expressing genes that may not be good for us, while blocking the expression of those that maintain health and youth.

SIRT6 affects glucose metabolism. As you have learned, increased blood sugar results in an increased production of insulin and a burst of inflammation. By helping to control levels of blood sugar, SIRT6 lowers the risk of developing diabetes, decreases body fat and the problems associated with obesity, and reduces the risk of heart disease and cancer.

Olive oil can activate SIRT6 better than other substances, such as the supplements fisetin and quercetin. Because SIRT6 is an enzyme dependent upon NAD, olive oil has been shown to be up to a hundred times more effective in increasing NAD—far more effective than any supplement on the market, on which sirtuin 6 is dependent. In addition, a promising substance found in seaweed called fucoidan may also upregulate SIRT6 and perhaps amplify the benefits.

Of the 7 human sirtuins, it appears that SIRT6 is the longevity protein that prevents aging in cells, tissues, and organs. Although the mechanisms underlying these effects are diverse, they all involve resistance to aging by promoting DNA damage repair, regulating glucose, and maintaining metabolic balance.

Activation of the sirtuins always affects the master metabolic regulator AMPK (the enzyme adenosine monophosphate-activated protein kinase) in a positive way. The first and most vital step in harnessing the power of the Beauty Molecule is learning how to activate AMPK. In the following chapter, I will take a deeper look at the master regulators AMPK and mTOR to explain how and why acetylcholine is the agent of beauty, health, and longevity.

4

THE BEAUTY MOLECULE
TRIGGERS THE MASTER
METABOLIC REGULATORS

SCIENTIFIC ADVANCES IN THE PAST 10 years have identified the molecular pathways and cell signals that can rejuvenate the body. We know now how to activate the metabolic switches that give us access to these pathways. Although we did not have this information 20 years ago, my anti-inflammatory diet included the right nutrients to affect those metabolic triggers. All the Perricone-recommended foods, full of omega-3s and polyphenols, will indirectly help to boost levels of the metabolic-regulator enzyme AMPK.

Our first and most vital step in harnessing the power of the Beauty Molecule is learning how to activate that master metabolic switch, AMPK, which regulates the intake and output of energy. By boosting production of the Beauty Molecule, acetylcholine, AMPK levels also will rise, because the Beauty Molecule upregulates AMPK.

Acting as an energy sensor within the cell, AMPK coordinates metabolic pathways and balances energy supply with energy demand. AMPK stimulates the metabolism, improves insulin sensitivity, decreases inflammation, and heightens muscle performance. Activation of AMPK may directly link to longevity.

My work has concentrated on strategies to enable cell repair and rejuvenation by reducing inflammatory damage. AMPK is a force for rejuvenation and has been a focus of my study for the past decade. One of the most important functions of the Beauty Molecule, acetylcholine, is that it activates AMPK. Once again, by stimulating synthesis of AMPK, the Beauty Molecule has a key role in an anti-aging process essential for good health.

Stimulating metabolism is a critical role. Metabolism consists of the chemical processes that occur within an organism to maintain life. The term "metabolism" is not just about how fast or slow we burn calories. To maintain life and preserve health, we must keep our metabolism normalized, in other words, balanced.

Acting as a molecular on/off switch, AMPK can induce cell growth and death, energy breakdown and storage, and can turn on specific genes for expression. Our cells are constantly adapting their metabolism to their environment, nutrient intake, and the need for energy. As an energy sensor, AMPK monitors the levels of the energy and storage molecule ATP (adenosine triphosphate), which is essential to life.

Produced in the mitochondria of cells, including the cells of the liver, brain, and muscles, and in fat cells, the AMPK molecule can sense if there are low levels of energy. In response, it will inhibit protein production to conserve energy. As the master switch, it reprograms cellular metabolism. AMPK affects glucose and fat metabolism and has a profound effect on removing older cells and their organelles. This process of moving the older cells is known as autophagy, and the removal of damaged mitochondria is mitophagy. Glucagon-like peptide-1 (GLP-1) and glucose-dependent insulinotropic polypeptide (GIP) are hormones that are secreted in our intestines when eating. These peptides result in secretion of insulin. As we will discuss in detail later in this book, GLP-1 and GIP receptors normalize blood sugar and metabolism and strongly upregulate AMPK. Pharmaceutical companies have synthesized these peptides to have a much longer half-life than the naturally occurring ones. These synthetic peptides, locking on to the receptor sites for GIP and GLP-1, are described as receptor agonists. When these receptors are activated, metabolism is normalized, appetite reduced, and a powerful anti-inflammatory effect results.

Scientists at the Salk Institute describe the metabolic enzyme AMPK as a "magic bullet" for health. Studies in animal models have shown that compounds that activate the enzyme have health-promoting effects to reverse diabetes, improve cardiovascular health, treat mitochondrial disease, and extend lifespan.

POLYPHENOLS ACTIVATE ACh AND AMPK

My background in nutrition motivates me to find foods that contribute to your beauty and longevity. I am talking about optimum health on a cellular level. Thanks to their acetylcholine and AMPK activity, polyphenol-rich foods have positive effects on mitochondrial biogenesis, metabolic processes, insulin sensitivity, and glucose uptake by the muscle tissue. There

FOODS THAT UPREGULATE AMPK

You are already familiar with a few of the foods that are rich in polyphenols. They are so important to your health and longevity that I list some of them again:

- Green tea
- Blackberries, strawberries, blueberries, raspberries
- Grapes
- Extra-virgin olive oil
- Cruciferous vegetables
- Spices such as cinnamon and turmeric
- Onions
- Dark chocolate
- Pomegranates

These foods help to alleviate stress on a cellular level and to maintain homeostasis. As polyphenol-rich foods help to control your appetite, they will increase muscle mass and decrease body fat.

are several foods that upregulate AMPK, improving the various metabolic pathways that will decrease insulin and inflammation. All the foods I recommend that are high in omega-3s and polyphenols are proven to decrease inflammation and to help to boost levels of AMPK. You will notice an increase and improvement in your energy levels as these foods upregulate the production of the Beauty Molecule and AMPK, normalizing energy production in the cell. These foods help us to alleviate stress on a cellular level while maintaining homeostasis. The foods I recommend also help to control appetite, increase muscle mass, and decrease body fat.

SUPPLEMENTS TO ACTIVATE AMPK

You can activate AMPK and balance your metabolism with supplements. Before taking new supplements, check with your healthcare provider and read the dosage instructions on the bottle. AMPK-activating supplements include:

- Alpha-lipoic acid
- Polyphenol antioxidants such as quercetin and EGCG, found in green tea
- Berberine
- Burdock root
- Dihydromyricetin
- Curcumin
- Red sage
- Zinc
- Omega-3 fish oil
- Apple cider vinegar
- Glucosamine
- Ginseng
- Carnitine

A CLOSE-UP OF CELL REJUVENATION

A young cell has optimal energy production. When that production diminishes, the aging process begins. Our bodies lose vitality as we age. The changes in our appearance, energy level, and mental acuity result from damage on a cellular level. The goal is to maximize cellular metabolism, which takes place in the mitochondria, converting chemical energy from food to energy in the body. To know how to rejuvenate cells, we need to understand the inner workings of mitochondria.

Mitochondria are often referred to as "cellular power plants." Converting food into fuel, these tiny furnaces are responsible for all energy production in the body. The mitochondria convert nutrients into hydrogen, which then enters the citric acid cycle, a metabolic pathway that connects carbohydrate, fat, and protein metabolism, within the mitochondria. Hydrogen is what fuels our bodies and makes it possible to create the energy storage and transfer molecule ATP, the energy currency for all cells. Without energy, the cell can no longer repair itself, which results in cellular breakdown and eventual organ failure. Healthy mitochondria are critical to slowing the aging process and keeping the body functioning at optimal health.

As you have read, free radicals cause cellular damage to substructures including the nucleus and other organelles. Free radicals can oxidize fats that make up the cell wall membrane and the membrane covering the mitochondria and the nucleus. This oxidation can lead to cellular dysfunction and serious damage to the immune system and major organs. It may surprise you to learn that some free radicals are generated in the mitochondria during the production of energy.

SENESCENCE: CELLULAR POWER FAILURE

A definition of senescence is the state of being old, the condition or process of deterioration with age. Senescence is aging on a cellular level. A senescent cell no longer has power to divide and grow. As we age, the number of pro-inflammatory senescent cells increases, activating an immunosuppressed state. When our immune system is suppressed, we lose our ability to fight infections and other diseases. Immunosuppression also prevents the clearance of senescent cells, resulting in accelerated aging and age-related diseases.

We must do everything we can to eliminate cells that become senescent, which can cause a decline in the function of all organs. This may include the loss of kidney function and poor performance of the cardiovascular system, as well as cognitive decline, loss of memory, and decrease in brain function.

Apoptosis, a genetically regulated form of cell death, occurs as a normal and controlled part of an organism's growth and development. This naturally occurring elimination process is vital for the removal of damaged cells. But not all cells that have lost their ability to divide are eliminated as they should be. Some of those senescent cells are not dormant. They remain active and secrete pro-inflammatory chemicals called cytokines and proteases, enzymes that break down proteins. These cells not only end up poisoning their environment and the cells directly associated with them, but also increase the inflammatory burden in the body, leading to a further decline of all organ systems.

The population of senescent cells that excrete these inflammatory chemicals are known as senescence-associated secretory phenotype (SASP). This form of cellular senescence turns senescent fibroblasts, a type of cell that contributes to the formation of connective tissue, into pro-inflammatory cells, which can promote tumor progression. Finding ways to eliminate senescent cells is an important focus in preventing aging and diseases like cancer.

The senescence response can be both tumor suppressive and carcinogenic, which scientists call a dual function. Biological processes like cellular senescence can be both beneficial and deleterious. Such dual effects are consistent with a major evolutionary theory of aging.

STRATEGIES FOR REMOVAL OF SENESCENT CELLS

One strategy for removing senescent cells is to use a variety of natural compounds found in high levels of polyphenol-rich foods that are abundant in the anti-inflammatory diet. Other methods include activating the body's elimination system via autophagy and mitophagy. Autophagy is a process that eliminates cells that are aged, defective, or damaged, while mitophagy clears out defective mitochondria.

Intracellular and extracellular stress can cause tremendous damage by slowly increasing a population of senescent cells that are either nonfunctional or secreting toxic products. This growth in senescent cell population is caused by mitochondrial deterioration and oxidative stress, when free radicals overwhelm the antioxidant system. A diet that is high in protein, good fats, rich antioxidants, and polyphenols is important for inhibiting an increase of senescent cells. Even with an excellent diet and lifestyle, supplemented with specific polyphenols and other antioxidants, the production of senescent cells will continue to move forward.

Scientists are very much interested in ways of removing these senescent cells. One area of research gaining tremendous traction is senolytics, which focuses on discovering agents that selectively eliminate senescent cells. The agents being studied include many different compounds, including certain drugs used in cancer treatment as well as polyphenolic compounds found in foods—the flavonoids fisetin and quercetin, for example. Fisetin is more powerful than quercitin, minus the potential risk of cancer drugs. A study published in *Aging* found that fisetin removed up to 70 percent of senescent cells without harming healthy, normal cells.

AUTOPHAGY TO THE RESCUE

Autophagy, a catabolic process, is a mechanism that can remove subcellular and cellular defects. Autophagy, which means "self-eating," refers to the elimination of an entire cell. The process involves the breakdown of the cell and the destruction of old, damaged, or abnormal proteins in the cytoplasm, the fluid inside the cell. The importance of autophagy cannot be overestimated because senescent cells accumulate with age, and their population must be reduced for continued health and longevity.

I came across an excellent metaphor to describe autophagy. Consider autophagy your body's cellular recycling system. It allows a cell to disassemble its junk parts and repurpose the salvageable bits and pieces into new, usable cell parts. A cell can discard the parts that are damaged or aged. Think of autophagy as quality control for your cells. An evolutionary self-preservation mechanism, autophagy can utilize parts of the cell needed for repair.

Mitophagy, another quality control mechanism, removes damaged mitochondria from a cell prior to cell death and inhibits mTOR, which blocks both mitophagy and autophagy. Mitophagy separates and isolates damaged mitochondria for removal. By degrading the damaged mitochondria, mitophagy helps to reinstate cellular balance. In ridding the body of senescent cells, autophagy and mitophagy reduce systemic inflammation.

mTOR is the opposite side of the balance. mTOR, which stands for mammalian target of rapamycin, is a protein kinase that regulates protein synthesis and cell growth in response to growth factors, nutrients, energy levels, and stress. An anabolic mechanism, mTOR creates muscle and other cells as it blocks mitophagy and autophagy.

The balance between the breaking-down, catabolic processes of autophagy and mitophagy, and the building, anabolic mTOR, is essential for maintaining robust health and youthful appearance. AMPK plays a role in maintaining that balance. When autophagy dominates, too many cells are removed, resulting in muscle loss, decreased bone density, and lusterless, wrinkled skin. The domination of mTOR means increased cell production, accumulation of senescent cells, and metabolic abnormalities in the body. mTOR is associated with cancer, arthritis, insulin resistance, and osteoporosis. As we age, autophagy diminishes, which results in an increased burden of senescent cells.

Protecting cells during times of cellular metabolic stress, AMPK promotes mitochondrial health. It maintains mitochondrial homeostasis or balance by stimulating autophagy and mitophagy and inhibiting mTOR. The balance is vital to cellular health. Mitochondrial homeostasis is an important longevity factor. Cells constantly need to manage their energy supply. We now know that the master regulator AMPK's effect on metabolism makes it possible to slow the aging process.

New science has shown that the Beauty Molecule promotes healthy cells and highly functioning mitochondria. In the subsequent pages and chapters, we will outline strategies to increase autophagy and mitophagy, both of which processes start the process of cellular rejuvenation.

FOODS TO TRIGGER CELL REPAIR

If you want to rejuvenate your cells, it can be as simple as eating foods that promote removal of senescent cells and damaged mitochondria. Here are just a few foods that trigger cell repair:

- Organic extra-virgin olive oil
- Cacao
- Curcumin
- Green tea
- Coffee
- Ginger
- Cinnamon
- Ginseng
- Garlic

At this point, you are familiar with many of the foods on this list. They each have a number of healing benefits. I list them for each of their functions to emphasize their healing power.

AMPK, METABOLIC DISEASE, AND EXERCISE

AMPK is important for effective interventions in many disease states. A good example is diabetes, the ultimate metabolic disease. The drug metformin was specifically designed for treatment of type 2 diabetes. Metformin has been found to activate AMPK in liver cells, which induces fatty acid oxidation, an increase in fat burning, and glucose uptake.

Metformin is receiving extensive attention as a potential anticancer treatment. Metformin-induced AMPK activation has also been shown to reduce cancer cell proliferation through several other mechanisms, including activation of c-Myc, HIF-1-alpha, and DICER1. There have been many studies showing improved survival rate in different cancer types for diabetic patients using metformin. The drug is gaining international interest for its potential use to prevent and treat different types of cancer, cardiovascular disease, aging, obesity, and neurological disorders. Data from in vitro and preclinical studies confirmed the anticancer activity of metformin against several types of cancer, which led to more than 55 clinical trials to investigate the potential anticancer effect against endometrial, prostate, pancreatic, lung, and breast cancer. Several systematic reviews have provided insight into the use of metformin for weight management and the treatment of obesity.

Metformin's mechanism of action is the upregulation of AMPK, which increases the uptake of blood sugar by muscle tissue and inhibits mTOR, the antagonist of AMPK activity. AMPK regulates metabolism and restores balance within the cell. AMPK functions in these separate ways: it inhibits the anabolic effects of mTOR and at the same time stimulates energy and promotes mitochondrial homeostasis.

By blocking mTOR, AMPK can be used to halt excess production of fats or fatty acids and be therapeutic in fatty liver disease. It also decreases blood glucose concentrations, in part due to enhanced muscle glucose uptake. Metformin has also been found to be extremely effective for nonalcoholic fatty liver disease, a predominant problem in the aging process. It is not surprising that it would be beneficial, because AMPK is produced in liver tissue.

In the 1960s, John Holloszy, the world's preeminent exercise biochemist/physiologist, discovered that physical endurance training produced higher mitochondrial levels, leading to increased glucose uptake by muscles. This process, called mitochondrial biogenesis, which occurs through the growth and division of preexisting mitochondria, is a direct response to the release of AMPK. As you know, one of AMPK's many functions is to promote the health and growth of mitochondria. Increased production of mitochondrial proteins and the fats needed for the mitochondrial membrane is necessary for mitochondrial biogenesis to take place.

Mitochondria form a complex, interconnected network within the cell center. Mitochondrial biogenesis helps the cell renew the mitochondrial network and improve mitochondrial function by slowing down the damage caused by mitochondrial dysfunction, a major contributor to aging.

One of the best ways to activate AMPK is to exercise. Exercise and muscle contraction stimulate the energy-generating process. When the Beauty Molecule, acetylcholine, is released during exercise, AMPK activation occurs at the neuromuscular junction.

Activation of AMPK is one of the main reasons exercise is one of my strategies, all of which are covered in part 2. When I recommend exercise, I do not mean hours in the gym. Though high-intensity exercise is effective, regular exercise—simply taking a daily walk, for example—is an AMPK activator.

A NOTE ON ALPHA-LIPOIC ACID, NEUROPATHY, AND NERVE GROWTH FACTOR

Alpha-lipoic acid, the universal metabolic antioxidant, has an indispensable role in normalizing metabolism. It acts to inhibit the action of acetylcholinesterase, the enzyme that blocks the production of the Beauty Molecule. Our goal is to increase levels of the Beauty Molecule, not reduce production.

Alpha-lipoic acid helps to control blood sugar and prevent the damage from excess blood sugar seen in diabetes. Peripheral neuropathy, a form of nerve damage, is associated with diabetes and high blood sugar. Peripheral nerves are those located outside the brain and spinal cord.

Peripheral neuropathy often causes weakness, numbness, and pain, most often in the hands and feet, though it can affect other areas and body functions. Motor neuropathy involves nerves that control muscles and movement. Neuropathy can also affect the autonomic nervous system, which controls involuntary systems in the body—for example, the heart and circulatory system, digestion, the bowels, and the bladder. Peripheral neuropathy usually begins with a tingling sensation in the legs and feet and sometimes the hand, indicating signs of damage to the nerves. That initial tingling can evolve to numbness, to degrees of chronic pain, to loss of sensation. Neuropathy associated with diabetes can lead to ulcers, which are open wounds or sores usually found on the bottom of the feet. Many of those with diabetic ulcers are hospitalized due to infections or other complications. In extreme cases, the infections require amputations.

Pathological pain or neuropathy is different from acute pain, which can be well controlled with treatments such as nonsteroidal anti-inflammatory drugs or opioids. Chronic pain is a common clinical problem that is poorly treated with available therapeutics. Most of the very few effective therapeutics available for pathological pain show limited efficacy.

A major clinical and public health problem, neuropathy affects nearly a third of the population of most developed countries and is responsible for enormous medical costs and loss of productivity in the workplace. With the global rise in diseases such as diabetes and the associated peripheral neuropathies, which can result in unrelenting pain, there is increasing emphasis on finding new therapeutic treatment for neuropathic pain.

Targeting AMPK activators could well signal a breakthrough in treating neuropathy. AMPK activators inhibit signaling pathways that are known to promote chronic pain. Alpha-lipoic acid increases acetylcholine levels, which in turn activates AMPK. Studies suggest that AMPK activators may be efficacious for the treatment of neuropathic pain and other chronic pain disorders. These studies found that AMPK activators can lead to a long-lasting reversal of pain hypersensitivity even long after treatment cessation.

Alpha-lipoic acid is used as a therapeutic treatment in Germany. In addition to its well-known activity as an antioxidant, its other properties include metabolic effects providing a wide range of beneficial effects on obesity-related conditions such as insulin resistance, metabolic syndrome, and type 2 diabetes, including their complications such as vascular damage. Alpha-lipoic acid can aid in liver detoxification, cardio-protection, insulin sensitivity improvement, and fat-burning capabilities. Alpha-lipoic acid also increases nerve growth factor, which assists in repairing damaged nerves.

A NOBEL-WORTHY DISCOVERY: NERVE GROWTH FACTOR

In 1986, Rita Levi-Montalcini, a brilliant Italian physician and scientist, was awarded the Nobel Prize in Physiology or Medicine, sharing the award with Stanley Cohen for their discoveries on nerve growth factors. Levi-Montalcini died aged 103 years, becoming the longest-living Nobel laureate, which, you will soon learn, is significant to her work.

Rita Levi-Montalcini contributed to our knowledge of the process of how we develop from a single cell, which divides to form new cells, which, in turn, divide and multiply as the process continues. Gradually different types of cells with different functions are formed.

In 1952 she isolated a substance harvested from tumors in mice that caused vigorous nervous system growth in chicken embryos. The discovery of what are now called growth factors provided a deeper understanding of medical problems like deformities, senile dementia, delayed wound healing, and tumor diseases.

This is where Dr. Levi-Montalcini's longevity comes into play. When discussing her work, she revealed that she had been using nerve growth factor in an ophthalmic solution that she placed in her eyes every day. The solution would then be carried to her brain. She strongly believed that the nerve growth factor eyedrops had enabled her to maintain the same neurological and cognitive function she enjoyed in her younger days well into her advanced years.

High levels of nerve growth factor can be found in individuals with conditions like arthritis, chronic headaches, and various generalized pain syndromes. With these conditions, the body produces nerve growth factor to repair the damaged nerves, relieving accompanying pain by reducing inflammation. AMPK activators have now been shown to alleviate pain in a broad variety of preclinical pain models, indicating that this mechanism might be engaged for the treatment of many types of pain. A key feature of the effect of AMPK activators in these models is that they can lead to a long-lasting reversal of pain hypersensitivity, even long after treatment cessation, indicative of disease modification.

To recap, the importance of AMPK cannot be overstated. AMPK activation promotes longevity. Research has found that AMPK, produced by acetylcholine, the Beauty Molecule, can fine-tune cell metabolism and increase your lifespan by up to 15 percent. AMPK ranks among the primary lines of defense against inflammation. It creates energy, inhibits mTOR, promotes autophagy and mitophagy, lowers blood sugar, normalizes weight, and heals the body.

Balance is a force at the systemic level as well. The following chapter delves into how the Beauty Molecule stimulates the autonomic nervous system to control inflammation.

5

THE BEAUTY MOLECULE STIMULATES AUTONOMIC BALANCE

THE LATEST RESEARCH GIVES US a view of what happens in the body when inflammation is unchecked. We have a new lens through which we can see how inflammation affects our body. Inflammation, the same bad actor, disrupts another well-documented pathway in our body: the autonomic nervous system. Inflammation alters and prevents the balance of the autonomic nervous system. To understand why maintaining this balance is so important, you need to be aware of how the nervous system functions.

BALANCE AND THE AUTONOMIC NERVOUS SYSTEM

We have two nervous systems that direct communication within the body by giving and receiving signals. The central nervous system consists of the brain and spinal cord. The peripheral nervous system includes all the nerves that branch out from the brain and spinal cord into other parts of the body. Part of the peripheral system, the autonomic nervous system, enables your body to function without any conscious effort on your part. Your internal organs operate on their own because of the autonomic nervous system. You breathe and digest automatically, and your heart beats on its own. The responsibilities of the autonomic nervous system are so significant that a large percent of the brain's output power is allotted to its function.

The autonomic nervous system is divided into two interacting, balancing systems. The sympathetic side activates the "fight or flight" arousal response, while the parasympathetic branch relies on "rest and digest" hormones. The sympathetic branch usually stimulates organs, while the parasympathetic slows down bodily processes. These systems work in opposition to regulate many functions and parts of the body.

When the sympathetic nervous system activates the fight-or-flight response, your body sets off a powerful series of reactions designed to help you survive a threatening situation. When you are frightened or stressed, your body releases hormones and neurotransmitters—adrenaline and cortisol, for example—that create a state of arousal and vigilance. Prepared for action, your body kicks into high gear: muscles tense, breathing becomes shallow and fast, the heart beats faster and more forcefully, blood pressure rises, skin pales, digestion stops. The response is hardwired into your brain to provide immediate protection from bodily harm.

The fight-or-flight response evolved to deal with short periods of physical stress. The problem is that emotional and psychological stress can set off the same emergency reaction. With chronic stress, the system meant to be a survival mechanism can itself become the threat. Activating the fight-or-flight response too often or for a sustained period can be damaging and can accelerate aging and disease. When fight-or-flight becomes a chronic state, an inflammatory cascade is set in motion.

Acting as a counterbalance to the emergency fight-or-flight response of the sympathetic nervous system, the parasympathetic creates a state of relaxation. The parasympathetic nervous system releases endorphins, dopamine, and serotonin to calm the body and quiet the fight-or-flight response. Endorphins boost your sense of well-being. Dopamine serves as an "incentivizer" to help you achieve your goal. Serotonin creates a relaxed and rested feeling. When the parasympathetic nervous system tilts the balance, blood pressure, heart rate, digestive function, and hormone levels return to normal. Inflammation levels fall. The chief neurotransmitter of the parasympathetic system is the Beauty Molecule, acetylcholine. Once again, the Beauty Molecule functions to tamp down inflammation.

Your autonomic system is in perfect balance when you are young and healthy. Your body calms down quickly after being in an aroused or anxious state. As you get older, you lose that equilibrium. Your autonomic nervous system is often turned on in the wrong direction and stays that way. When rest-and-digest is no longer our baseline, sympathetic arousal dominates. Living in a prolonged or chronic state of fight-or-flight high alert increases inflammation and metabolic dysfunction that lead to cellular aging, disease, and decreased health span, all of which are evident in your appearance. The Beauty Molecule's stimulation of the parasympathetic nervous system reduces inflammation on a cellular level, producing radiance in the skin.

A study of 1,882 participants is described in the paper "Autonomic Imbalance as a Predictor of Metabolic Risks, Cardiovascular Disease, Diabetes, and Mortality." The goal of the study was to identify early predictors of metabolic disorders, cardiovascular disease, diabetes, and early mortality. The study found that each of these diseases was directly connected to autonomic system imbalance. The study noted that hyperinsulinemia, as high blood sugar is called, increases sympathetic nervous system activity. The paper went on to describe autonomic imbalance as excessive sympathetic activity and too little parasympathetic activity.

Restoring equilibrium to the autonomic nervous system allows the body to function optimally.

FLIPPING THE REST-AND-DIGEST SWITCH

My belief in the power of meditation and its effect on the autonomic nervous system has been confirmed by wonderful stories from people eager to share their transformative experiences. Andy's story is no exception. I am very happy to share it with you.

As Andy explained, it all started when he came down with COVID in February 2020 at the start of the pandemic. By May of 2020 it had become what is known as long COVID. Since May 2021, he was perhaps 80 percent cured. It was a long haul, but Andy said that meditation's effect on inflammation contributed a lot to his healing. He wanted to share his story in hopes that it can give others faith in their ability to get their parasympathetic nervous system in gear to tamp down inflammation.

Andy reported that his COVID symptoms were very mild, but so strange they didn't appear on the CDC list until late 2020. He experienced fatigue, breathlessness from minor exertion, fevers, and intense dizziness every time he bent over.

Unfortunately, his long COVID symptoms increased and intensified. Heat flashes, panic attacks, tachycardia (an abnormally rapid heartbeat), relentless chronic fatigue, acid reflux, mucus attacks, and the fear of passing out on the street had turned him almost completely into a shut-in. To make matters worse, he had no idea what was triggering any of this.

After seven months, Andy was able to join Mount Sinai Hospital's long COVID group, which had a lengthy waiting list. It was here that he met two physicians who offered some clues as to what was happening to him. The first doctor told him that his chronic fatigue was different from the classic version seen in Lyme patients, because his sleep was restful and exercise didn't cause a relapse.

A second doctor pointed out that eating big, carbohydrate-heavy meals might be triggering the tachycardia. The breathlessness inspired Andy to turn to Mount Sinai's recommended breathing program, Stasis (https://www.stasis.life). He began using the only available chronic fatigue therapy, a low-dose naltrexone, usually used to block opioid receptors in the nervous system. He started to meditate with the goal of getting more effective rest so that he might not need to nap every 90 minutes or so. One deep meditation revealed a pounding heart, lungs forgetting to breathe, and a relentless surging, like a body fighting for its life.

A couple of weeks later, Andy reported that he had wolfed down a small pizza. He was not surprised when he experienced an immediate doubling of his heart rate, explosive acid reflux, and an all-out panic attack. It was at this point he recognized that he needed a major dietary overhaul.

Andy had heard of Dr. Perricone and the anti-inflammatory diet. He loved fish, especially salmon, and who doesn't love the crisp salads and sweet fresh berries that Dr. Perricone championed? He also cut out refined and processed foods, and by dropping those inflammatory foods, his meal size was immediately decreased. Bye-bye huge plate of greasy fries smothered in ketchup. No more Happy Meals—a misnomer if ever there was one. Fast-forward 3 days, and Andy was dramatically improved.

He said that the speed of his recovery might have been a coincidence. Those who previously had long-haul symptoms from COVID, Epstein-Barr, and other viral infections reported getting well or significantly better at the one-year mark, and he had just hit the one-year mark. He still had various problems, including mild chronic fatigue and not-so-mild depression, which he learned to treat successfully with meditation and breath work.

At this point, Andy began to research the relationship between the immune, endocrine, and nervous systems. His problem turned out to be dysautonomia, a condition in which the sympathetic nervous system is revved up, setting off the fight-or-flight response. Now that he had identified what was happening, Andy began to study the autonomic nervous system—the sympathetic and parasympathetic systems—in search of therapies for stimulating the parasympathetic nervous system, known as the firefighter's cure, or vagus nerve triggering. Understanding how the vagus nerve functioned to fight inflammation was the first time his symptoms made sense. Andy could see that the effects of meditating and breath work worked for him because they calmed down his overactive, inflamed autonomic nervous system.

Andy firmly believed that the anti-inflammatory diet rounded out the picture on his road to recovery, giving him a tremendous edge in eliminating the frightening symptoms. With anti-inflammatory foods, Andy's body could catch up to the mental serenity the meditation and breath work induced. It was a perfect combination to get mind/body/spirit in sync. As we know, this is a very real problem facing all of us in today's world. As Andy said, it was vitally important to look at the big picture, and diet is as critical as the mental/spiritual elements.

Andy said that though it might sound "New Agey," after being sick for fifteen months, he was desperate for solutions. He wanted to give up many times but persevered. He is delighted to be able to report that he is not only himself again, he is a better, calmer self, and now has his life back. The food choices, deep breathing, and meditation were significant components of Andy's healing. He is firmly convinced that he would not be this well or happy if any one of these components had not been a major part of his therapy. Andy is now study-ing and teaching meditation and breath work, and the anti-inflammatory diet is a major cornerstone of his new life. It was gratifying to receive Andy's per-sonal thanks and his belief that he could not have gotten to his new and im-proved state without following the Perricone recommendations.

Andy's story is not unique, but it is heartening. If people only realized how the anti-inflammatory lifestyle and meditation create the ideal en-vironment for mental and physical well-being, they would be lining up to learn more. Sometimes it takes a frightening experience to serve as a wake-up call to take control of our lives. In Andy's case, the COVID expe-rience was not without its silver lining.

THE VAGUS NERVE TRIGGERS AN ANTI-INFLAMMATORY, RELAXATION RESPONSE

The vagus nerve is the major parasympathetic nerve. Vagus means "wander-ing," which refers to the fact that the nerve extends from the brain stem down the neck and into the chest and abdomen. It is the longest and most complex of the 12 pairs of cranial nerves that originate from the brain stem. The vagus nerve controls the functioning of the most significant organs of your body. It stimulates the heart, major blood vessels, airways, lungs, esophagus, stomach, and intestines. Triggering a relaxation response, the vagus nerve is responsible for decreasing alertness, blood pressure, and heart rate as it promotes calm, relaxation, and digestion. In addition, the vagus nerve fights inflammation by sending an anti-inflammatory signal to the rest of the body. Our goal is to activate the vagus nerve and the parasympathetic nervous system.

THE MULTITASKING VAGUS NERVE

The functions of the vagus nerve affect the entire body, and the Beauty Molecule triggers the vagus nerve. In addition to regulating the parasym-pathetic and sympathetic nervous system, the vagus nerve signals:

- The respiratory system to affect our rate of breathing
- The cardiovascular system by dilating and constricting blood vessels, which affects blood pressure, decreasing or increasing heart rate and heart muscle contractions
- The pupils to dilate or constrict
- The urinary tract to increase or decrease bladder capacity
- The digestive system to increase or decrease digestive contractions, known as peristalsis or gastric motility
- To correct autonomic imbalance, lessening the risk of metabolic disorders
- To affect our alertness or cognition. The elevation of the Beauty Molecule enhances cognition.

THE ICEMAN COMETH

Wim Hof, also known as the Iceman, is a Dutch motivational speaker and extreme athlete noted for his ability to withstand low temperatures. He has become famous for a variety of unusual and extreme activities. When he injects himself with bacterial toxin, he does not get the expected severe reaction of prolonged shaking, chills, and fever, which would cause him to be bedridden for a few days. He manages to avoid this outcome by somehow activating or deactivating his immune system through acetylcholine. And that's where we find the big disconnect.

Using a variety of methodologies including MRIs, the scientists studying this phenomenon have concluded that Hof avoids these reactions largely through the sympathetic nervous system. I disagree with this hypothesis. I am convinced that Wim Hof's body resists the injected bacteria mainly through the parasympathetic nervous system, with less participation of the sympathetic nervous system. I believe that Hof's body accomplished this surprising immunity by secreting acetylcholine, the Beauty Molecule, which attaches to a nicotinic receptor on the white blood cells, blocking the cytokine storm that would normally be set in motion under these extreme circumstances.

Hof's techniques consist of a combination of frequent cold exposure, breathing techniques, and meditation to increase the amount of oxygen in his body. One of his techniques involves deep breathing, which activates the vagus nerve, also called the X cranial nerve or tenth cranial nerve, the longest and most complex of the cranial nerves. The areas of his brain his techniques access are visible on PET scans.

When he hyperventilates, he activates an evolutionary process, one that our ancient ancestors experienced in stressful situations, such as running away from a saber-toothed tiger, the fight-or-flight response. The hyperventilation triggers activation of the sympathetic nervous system. Rather than relying on fear or stress to trigger the emergency response, Wim Hof can do it on demand.

When he implements his technique, he must be activating the Beauty Molecule and the parasympathetic nervous system, because he is mitigating the inflammatory immune response that might otherwise come from bacterial toxin. By attaching to the nicotinic receptor, the Beauty Molecule tones down the secretion of cytokines.

. . . .

Today we know how to restore balance in the autonomic nervous system. This discovery is one of the main reasons I decided to write this book. Once again, it is the result of control of cellular inflammation. When inflammation disrupts the cell's normal biochemical functions, all organ systems, including the autonomic nervous system, are affected.

The primary neurotransmitter of the parasympathetic nervous system, the Beauty Molecule, acetylcholine, is responsible for cueing that part of the autonomic nervous system to increase activity. Not only does the Beauty Molecule stimulate the production of the rest-and-digest hormones, but it also inhibits the immune system from excessive production of inflammatory cytokines. With the knowledge of how to use the Beauty Molecule to restore balance in the autonomic nervous system, we have discovered another path to optimal health and glowing beauty.

WHAT YOU CAN DO TO TURN ON YOUR PARASYMPATHETIC NERVOUS SYSTEM

There are many techniques for jump-starting your parasympathetic nervous system. Part 2 of this book explains several strategies for stimulating the inflammation-fighting rest-and-digest parasympathetic system. Here are some of the actions you can take to restore balance in your autonomic nervous system:

- Deep breathing
- Humming, singing, chanting, or gargling
- Laughter
- Meditation
- Positive social connections
- Hugging
- Massage—especially reflexology
- Yoga, tai chi
- Cold showers (for at least 30 seconds)
- Prayer
- Probiotics
- Omega-3 supplements
- Exercise

As you can see, these actions are not very challenging. The vagus nerve's response to any one of them will relax you and lower inflammation in your body.

VAGAL TONE

The higher the tone of your vagus nerve, the more efficient your body is in activating the parasympathetic nervous system. Increasing vagal tone is an important goal. Heart rate variability is one way to measure vagal tone. As you breathe in, your heart rate speeds up a bit. As you breathe out, your heart slows down a little. Your vagal tone is measured by the difference between your inhalation and exhalation heart rates. The higher the tone, the better you are at relaxing.

This balance between the parasympathetic and sympathetic nervous systems is extremely important for maintaining homeostasis in all the cells of the body. Homeostasis is critical to health and longevity. A simple test done in a doctor's office can give great insight into how well or how poorly this balance is maintained. The test measures heart rate variability, which is the variation, in milliseconds, between consecutive heartbeats. The test measures fluctuations between each heartbeat. Detectable only with specialized devices, these fluctuations indicate current or future health problems, including heart conditions and mental health issues like anxiety and depression.

When we inhale, the autonomic nervous system is responsible for a slight increase in heart rate. As we exhale, a slight decrease in heart rate occurs. By measuring this difference between your inhalation and exhalation heart rates, the physician can then identify your heart rate variability. In fact, it is such an accurate test that we could predict our longevity based upon heart rate variability.

THE CHOLINERGIC SYSTEM

The Beauty Molecule, acetylcholine, works through the vagus nerve, which reaches into major organs, including the liver, heart, spleen, and gastrointestinal tract. Stress and fatigue can inflame this nerve. Rather than expanding on the outside forces that affect this nerve, we focus in on what influences the function of the vagus nerve on the cellular level. When injury, pathogens, or danger to tissue is present, an automatic molecular response in our cells, activated by cellular sensors, kicks in.

The Beauty Molecule is at the core of the cholinergic system, which is composed of organized nerve cells that use acetylcholine in the transduction or conversion of action potentials. These nerve cells are activated by, or contain and release, acetylcholine during the propagation of a nerve impulse. In the cholinergic pathway, the vagus nerve carries efferent, or outgoing, signals from the brain via acetylcholine to regulate the innate immune response to injury, pathogens, or tissue damage. In addition, the vagus nerve carries signals from the gastrointestinal tract via afferent, or incoming, signals to activate the mind-gut connection. Afferent neurons carry information from sensory receptors of the skin and other organs to the central nervous system, while efferent neurons carry outgoing information away from the brain and spinal cord to the muscles and glands of the body.

As you have learned, the Beauty Molecule, acetylcholine, can activate either the parasympathetic or sympathetic nervous systems, depending on whether the desired result is to increase or relax activity. For example, acetylcholine signals both the sympathetic and parasympathetic nervous system in the gastric system, depending on whether the result is to increase or decrease activity in the gut.

The cholinergic pathway can be activated to increase or decrease production of the Beauty Molecule to bring balance to the autonomic system, overcoming problems that occur when the autonomic system is out of balance. Those conditions include trauma, stress reactions, and post-traumatic stress disease. Acetylcholine has shown promising results addressing obesity, a condition that results in autonomic imbalance and leads to an increased risk of metabolic disorders and mitochondrial dysfunction.

The Beauty Molecule works systemically to maintain balance in the autonomic nervous system by helping to fight inflammation caused by the immune response. This action has an immeasurable impact on your health and well-being.

I am excited to tell you about my latest discovery and a new inflammation fighter now available to everyone. The following chapter covers my recent research on hydrogen as a powerful antidote to health-destroying inflammation.

6

THE MAGIC BULLET HYDROGEN: SMALL BUT MIGHTY

PRACTICING MEDICINE HAS BEEN BOTH a passion and a joy for many decades. My greatest love is research—searching for that elusive answer to curing our ills, keeping us healthy longer, lengthening our lifespan, and keeping the *joie* in the *joie de vivre*, the antidote to the chronic subclinical inflammation occurring on a cellular level, invisible to the naked eye but deadly just the same. Antioxidant-rich foods and supplements and topicals, especially those that trigger the release of the Beauty Molecule, are indispensable therapeutics. Only relatively recently in my decades-long quest for the magic bullet have I learned of a substance that meets my criteria. My criteria are nontoxic, affordable, and available. Previous research is littered with "magic bullets," often hyped but rarely living up to the claims. These substances are promising, but they do not deliver. Resveratrol is an example. Resveratrol, found in the skin of grapes, blueberries, and raspberries, is a powerful polyphenol with many superior health benefits. The hope had been that resveratrol could extend the human lifespan, but that has since been disproven.

LIGHTNING STRIKES

As I was paging through a copy of the science journal *Nature Medicine*, I came across an article that discussed the benefits of the anti-inflammatory capabilities of hydrogen and its impact on health. Atomic hydrogen is the smallest and the first element on the periodic table. Hydrogen, an unstable atom, exists naturally only as molecular hydrogen, called H_2. Molecular hydrogen is a gas that is colorless, odorless, tasteless, and flammable. Until a decade ago, hydrogen was thought to be completely inert, having no activity in the body. I was about to discover that hydrogen was anything but inert.

Intrigued by the article I stumbled on, I decided to look into hydrogen to see what the science had to say. Many studies of various animal models examined effects of the inhalation of hydrogen gas or drinking hydrogen-infused water. There was not much research done in the area of human medicine. At first, I was skeptical that hydrogen could have any interaction in the body.

Studies have since shown that hydrogen inhalation therapy can help patients who have suffered cardiac arrest, by reducing damage to brain functions and heart muscle tissue. In China and Japan, inhaling hydrogen gas for increased vitality and well-being is common practice. I soon learned that water infused with hydrogen has long been available in the mass market in Japan, where the majority of the studies on hydrogen's efficacy originate.

I was intrigued that Asians have recognized for some time that increasing hydrogen intake exerts a powerful anti-inflammatory effect. I realized that we too may have discovered a powerful, nontoxic substance to add to our inventory of viable therapeutics.

Scientists then discovered that when hydrogen is administered to living cells, it has a powerful antioxidant and anti-inflammatory effect. Hydrogen targets and neutralizes the most dangerous and destructive free radicals, the reactive oxygen species (ROS). The toxic hydroxyl radical causes significant damage to cell structures and contributes to their functional decline; in other words, aging. These ROS launch their cycle of destruction by stealing electrons from molecules in DNA, proteins, and fats, setting off the oxidative stress chain reaction. H_2 gives up electrons to ROS free radicals, which stabilizes them and stops their destructive course.

The specificity of hydrogen's target is very important, because mild reactive oxygen species are an essential part of normal cell signaling and functioning. Hydrogen is a smart antioxidant because it specifically targets the strong and dangerous ROS like the hydroxyl radical and allows the mild ROS to function.

Indiscriminately treating cells with strong antioxidants can interfere with normal cell function. The good news is that hydrogen is the ultimate smart molecule, because it can rapidly penetrate all tissue cells and subcellular components such as the mitochondria and the nucleus. Researchers have discovered that its size makes molecular hydrogen, the tiniest molecule in existence, highly bioavailable to cells.

Unlike other antioxidants like CoQ10, the hydrogen molecule is both fat and water soluble, which enables it to be delivered to the highly lipid membranes of the cells and organelles. Hydrogen can pass through the blood-brain barrier to exert positive effects. Hydrogen water has great benefit to the skin, illustrating the brain-beauty connection once again.

HYDROGEN IN ACTION

Thanks to the hydrogen science advocates in Asia, several hundred studies have been conducted in medical research facilities and academia that demonstrate that the benefits of hydrogen therapy are diverse and cover many metabolic and aging-related disorders. More than 400 studies, including at least 30 human studies, have shown that molecular hydrogen is therapeutic in every organ of the body and against more than 140 diseases, including metabolic syndrome, diabetes, obesity, atherosclerosis, and several cancers.

H$_2$, THE SMART MOLECULE

Hydrogen targets and neutralizes the strongest and most dangerous free radicals.

Hydrogen can rapidly penetrate all tissue cells and subcellular components such as the mitochondria and the nucleus. Researchers have discovered that its size makes molecular hydrogen, the tiniest molecule in existence, highly bioavailable to cells. Hydrogen further benefits the body in these broad ways:

- Converts toxic hydroxyl radicals to water in the body
- Hydrogen water mimics fasting and exercise (to be discussed in part 2) by turning on and activating AMPK, the metabolic switch.
- Has a beneficial effect on cell signaling, cell metabolism, and gene expression, with anti-inflammatory, anti-obesity, and anti-aging results
- Suppresses cytokines, the proteins involved in inflammation, and turns on mechanisms that protect against cell death
- Hydrogen is important to gut health. Hydrogen-rich water intake induced a significant increase in the abundance of lactobacillus, ruminococcus, and clostridium XI, the healthful gut bacteria that aid your digestion and have other anti-aging benefits. This matters because, as the intestinal microbiota changes with aging, an imbalance in intestinal microorganisms can lead to many age-related degenerative diseases and unhealthy aging. The gut microbiome is now being considered as a key factor in the aging process.
- Studies have found that hydrogen-rich water induced protection of the gut barrier integrity and upregulation of butyrate-producing bacteria. Butyrate is produced when "good" bacteria in your gut help your body break down dietary fiber in your colon.
- Drinking hydrogen water is an ideal strategy for improving digestion, because aging can slow gut motility and weaken the immune system. New medications introduced to your body to combat age-related diseases could destroy necessary bacteria in your gut microbiome.
- H$_2$ has proven to have a beneficial effect on aging skin.

Knowing that hydrogen-enriched water can reverse skin aging and have a therapeutic effect on so many illnesses—the epidemics of our time—has motivated me to make this natural cure accessible to everyone. Just as salmon and blueberries are foods I have championed for decades, I am delighted to report that hydrogen water is just as vital for everyone wishing to retain youthful vigor and radiance. We cannot stop the clock yet, but we can certainly slow it down considerably by adding hydrogen water to an anti-inflammatory diet.

Although drinking any type of purified water will hydrate you and improve your skin tone, hydrogen water does so much more. In addition to drinking hydrogen water three times a day, also continue with drinking ample pure water every day. Hydrogen water is an important and transformative addition to a health- and beauty-focused lifestyle.

FURTHER BENEFITS OF HYDROGEN WATER

The sweeping, health-enhancing benefits of drinking hydrogen water include:

- Reducing fatigue/increasing energy by boosting levels of NAD and NADH, which are critical to mitochondrial energy production
- Enhancing nutrient absorption
- Removing toxins
- Improving muscle tone
- Improving joint mobility
- Speeding recovery from workouts
- Reducing skin aging
- Increasing skin radiance within 3 days in the same manner as the 3-day anti-inflammatory diet
- Improving blood circulation
- Aiding in healthful cholesterol levels
- Protecting cells to retard aging
- Combating jet lag
- Combating the toxic effects of alcohol, alleviating hangovers

Hydrogen should be an important adjunct on your travels, as it will rapidly alleviate travel fatigue. H_2 is an absolute must for combating jet lag when changing time zones. It has also been shown to be an efficacious remedy for hangovers—although the best remedy is prevention by drinking in moderation in the first place.

I was so inspired by studies of the positive effects of hydrogen water that I traveled to Japan to meet with their leading scientists. I have since introduced a treatment here in the United States. As you know, a young cell is characterized by its energy production, and that critical energy production greatly diminishes with age. The ability of hydrogen to store and transport energy makes it indispensable for cell rejuvenation.

HYDROGEN, ENERGY, AND THE MITOCHONDRIA

In 1937, the Nobel Prize in Physiology or Medicine was awarded to Albert von Szent-Györgyi de Nagyrápolt, a brilliant physician and scientist, for his discoveries in connection with the energy-producing processes, focusing on the role of vitamin C in the efficient use of carbohydrates, fats, and proteins.

Prior to his groundbreaking research, science lacked knowledge of basic nutrition. Scurvy, the result of vitamin C deficiency, was among many diseases caused by malnutrition. His discovery laid the foundation for modern nutrition.

Because vitamin C, ascorbic acid, is by far the best known and most popular nutritional supplement in a vast pantheon of supplements, it is easy to take its importance for granted. Vitamin C is not only a powerful antioxidant, which neutralizes the destructive effects of free radicals, but it also is essential to the growth and health of bones, teeth, gums, ligaments, and blood vessels. Vitamin C plays a key role in the formation of collagen, the body's major building protein, and is essential to the proper functioning of all internal organs as well as the health of the skin.

I include Professor Szent-Györgyi in this hydrogen chapter because his acceptance speech for the Nobel Prize focused on the energy-providing role of hydrogen. Although the Nobel Prize was given to Professor Szent-Györgyi for his elucidation of the structure of vitamin C, the Karolinska Institute, presenting the award, explained that his work discovered the path of energy production in the cell. Szent-Györgyi went on to identify and study actin and myosin, proteins responsible for muscle contraction, and demonstrated that the compound adenosine triphosphate (ATP) is the immediate source of energy necessary for muscle contraction. His remarkable work laid the foundation for Sir Hans Krebs's explanation of what later would be known as the Krebs cycle: the three-stage process by which living cells break down organic molecules in the presence of oxygen to harvest the energy required for growth and division. Relentless in his pursuit of that path, Szent-Györgyi is responsible for much of what we know today about energy production in the mitochondria.

His acceptance speech for the Nobel Prize reflected his fascination with the function of hydrogen's interaction with oxygen to produce energy:

> Our body really only knows one fuel, hydrogen. The foodstuff, carbohydrate, is essentially a packet of hydrogen, a hydrogen supplier, a hydrogen donor, and the main event during its combustion is the splitting off of hydrogen. The combustion of hydrogen is the real energy-supplying reaction. To the elucidation of reaction, which seems so simple, I have devoted all my energy for the last fifteen years.

Today we know that hydrogen is essential for producing ATP in the electron transport chain. The primary tasks of the last stage of the electron transport chain are to transfer energy from the electron carriers to even more ATP molecules, which are the "batteries" that power work within the mitochondria, and to upregulate the sirtuin enzymes, introduced in chapter 3. Sirtuins function to normalize metabolism and maintain DNA structure and all forms of homeostasis within the cells. Sirtuins are activated when hydrogen increases levels of NAD. Increasing NAD levels to activate sirtuins for cellular repair is one of the best anti-aging strategies we have to date.

PUTTING HYDROGEN TO THE TEST

In my role as researcher, I was interested to see if I could replicate the Japanese studies, using the same methodologies that demonstrated hydrogen's anti-inflammatory activity. In more than one instance, I did not get the positive results being published. Armed with the information I had gathered in Japan, I was eager to do my own study on hydrogen water. One of the benefits offered by the commercial and scientific promotion of hydrogen water is access to more energy. That very interesting premise seemed an excellent place to start my own research.

I consulted with my friend and colleague Dr. Peter Pugliese to look into the benefits of hydrogen. I explained that I was seeking a method that would allow me to quantify changes in energy levels in the body to prove that hydrogen increases energy in the cells. Dr. Pugliese, a brilliant scientist, physician, and fellow researcher, told me that he might have an idea. Energy is produced in the mitochondria in what is known as the tricarboxylic acid (TCA) cycle, also referred to as the Krebs or citric acid cycle, the main source of energy for cells. Hydrogen, active in producing energy, is one of the key molecules in the Krebs cycle.

Peter explained that the skin is rich in NADH, which is the donor of hydrogen becoming NAD after the hydrogen is handed off to the Krebs cycle. NAD cycles and picks up hydrogen from our food and regenerates NADH once again. In a series of enzymatic reactions, the TCA cycle generates the reducing equivalents NADH and $FADH_2$, required to transfer electrons to the mitochondrial respiratory chain, also known as the electron transport chain. The primary task of the last stage of the electron transport chain is to transfer energy from the electron carriers to even more ATP molecules.

NADH is the one molecule in the skin that fluoresces, which means that it emits light or another type of radiation. Dr. Pugliese suggested using a light frequency on the skin that would excite NADH, alerting us to the NADH level in the skin. The light frequency would send back a signal that we could read with a computer, allowing us to measure this energy molecule in a noninvasive manner.

Our next step was to implement a formal study to establish a baseline measure of NADH, using the apparatus that Dr. Pugliese suggested. The participating subjects wore an LED light strapped onto their arm to measure NADH levels. Once the baseline of NADH level in the skin was established, we could observe in real time any subsequent increases in NADH through the computer. We were delighted to observe that the NADH levels began to show an increase within 2 minutes of drinking the hydrogen water. At the end of 15 minutes, a 12.5 percent increase of NADH occurred in the majority of subjects being tested. This increase demonstrates that the tiny hydrogen molecule entered the mitochondria portion of the cell, which produces energy. As hydrogen is the smallest element on the periodic table, hydrogen gas dissolved in water can rapidly diffuse throughout the body in a matter of a few minutes, entering the cells, including the mitochondria, to increase the levels of NADH.

This study proved to me that hydrogen can and does increase cellular energy. The finding inspired me to pursue the production of high-quality hydrogen water previously unavailable to the general population in therapeutic levels.

Young cells are characterized by high energy, and energy is needed for uptake of nutrients, expelling waste and carrying on structural repair. Old cells have low energy, poor repair, and their ability to utilize nutrients and remove waste is compromised. Hydrogen powers and recharges cells, returning them to a more youthful level by restoring the cells' diminished ability to ingest nutrients, remove waste more efficiently, and repair damage, all of which add up to the reversal of the aging process.

HYDROGEN AND METABOLIC SYNDROME

One of hydrogen's key benefits, as shown in many studies, is the normalization of our metabolism. As we age, one of the biggest killers is the loss of metabolic control, which is seen as an increase in blood sugar, despite an increase in insulin.

This change is called metabolic syndrome. A growing problem in our society, metabolic syndrome is associated with increased blood pressure, high blood sugar, excess body fat around the waist, and abnormal cholesterol or triglyceride levels. A protruding abdomen is an indicator of abdominal fat, which is one of the biggest risk factors for metabolic syndrome. Metabolic syndrome increases the risk for heart disease, diabetes, and stroke. These metabolic changes also put us at risk for cognitive decline. Metabolic syndrome is closely linked to overweight or obesity and inactivity, as well as to a condition called insulin resistance.

With insulin resistance, even if insulin levels are adequate, blood sugar does not go down to a normal level. To identify insulin resistance, doctors look for impaired fasting blood glucose, which is a level higher than 100 on a blood glucose test.

NADH and its partner NAD have profound effects on metabolism. There are a number of products on the market currently that will increase levels of NAD and help normalize metabolism. Proven to increase levels of NADH and NAD, hydrogen is probably the best and most efficient way to increase these levels, rather than paying for expensive supplement products like NMN (niacinamide mononucleotide) and niacinamide riboside.

Dr. Tyler LeBaron, the founder of the Molecular Hydrogen Institute, ran an excellent double-blind, placebo-controlled study. The study was conducted on 60 subjects over a period of 24 weeks. These 60 participants were chosen because they were diagnosed with metabolic syndrome. They were divided into two groups of 30 in this double-blind study. One group received the active hydrogen water, the other group plain water. At the end of the 24 weeks all of the subjects who received hydrogen water showed marked improvement in the metabolic tests, and they could no longer be categorized as having metabolic syndrome. The plain water (placebo) group showed no improvement in this study. If we can halt metabolic syndrome by drinking hydrogen water in the general population, we can extend lives and dramatically lower healthcare costs. The true miracle of drinking hydrogen water is that it prevents the downstream problems of all of the major Western diseases including diabetes, heart disease, and neurological decline. An added benefit is that there was an average weight loss of 8 pounds without any other change to diet. It is also hepatoprotective (preventing damage to the liver) and also protective of kidney function.

HYDROGEN WATER–CHOOSE WISELY

If you plan to introduce hydrogen water into your daily routine, choose your product with care. Hydrogen must be present in the water in adequate levels to have the therapeutic effects I have mentioned. Experts agree that 0.8 parts per million is the lowest acceptable level of H_2 for therapeutic benefits. More than 1 part per million is the ideal level required to achieve optimal benefits.

Hydrogen dissipates very quickly because it is such a small molecule. Keep this in mind when considering the packaging, because hydrogen water will diffuse right through the container when packaged in plastic or glass. My studies have found that aluminum cans with a polymer lining are the best way to maintain therapeutic levels. We have seen that correctly manufactured cans maintain 1.2 parts per million for more than 6 years. Beware of any container that is not a sealed can, such as a pouch, because when tested they have subtherapeutic levels. Once the can is open, I recommend that you drink the entire contents within 10 minutes. To maintain optimum hydrogen levels, do not pour the water into a glass or use a straw.

Although this might be the first time you are hearing about hydrogen-infused water, it is readily available online. My hydrogen-infused water, Dr. Perricone Hydrogen Water, is packaged in aluminum cans. Hydrogen tablets, which you can add to pure water, are an option. Hydrogen-producing water bottles can be found for a wide range of prices, but make sure they produce a high enough level of hydrogen to be therapeutic.

For overall health and well-being, disease prevention, and a superior energy boost, hydrogen water is hard to beat.

7

BRINGING IT ALL BACK HOME: NEUROCEUTICALS, THE BEAUTY MOLECULE, AND THE BRAIN-BEAUTY CONNECTION

RECENTLY I HAD THE HONOR of being the keynote speaker chosen to address a large group of leading cosmetic scientists in New York City. Imagine my surprise when I discovered that the main topic of conversation was the emerging field of neurocosmetics. Perricone readers are well aware of my pioneering work in what I call the brain-beauty connection. I have spent more than two decades studying this vital relationship and devising neuroceuticals, topical formulations, and nutritional and lifestyle strategies to enhance all of its exciting aspects. I was dumbfounded to discover that this important tenet of my teaching and writings was suddenly "new." As the rest of the world catches up, I have decided the time is right to reintroduce this fascinating connection, a connection at the very cornerstone of my lifetime of study and research.

UNDERSTANDING EMBRYONIC DEVELOPMENT

To recap the brain-beauty connection for this discussion of neuroceuticals, let me explain the close connection between the skin and the brain and the key role that neuropeptides play. Neuropeptides are tiny strings of amino acids found naturally in our bodies. These neuropeptides control biological function. They are active in the brain and the skin. The intimate relationship of neuropeptides with the skin begins in the embryonic state as human life forms.

We begin our development in the womb as an embryo. Embryonic stem cells are cells with the potential to develop into many different types of cells in the body. In the embryo, these stem cells are made up of three layers of tissue. One of the layers, known as the ectoderm, is responsible for producing all the characteristics of the skin, hair, and nails. They are also responsible for brain cell development. Derived from the same level of tissue, skin and brain cells are closely related. I call this relation the brain-beauty connection. This knowledge has led me to make many discoveries in skin rejuvenation.

This direct link—the brain-beauty connection—is even more evident in the connection between the brain and the action of nerves in the skin. The skin contains abundant nerve endings, which provide information to the brain.

The skin is composed of many different types of cells, such as fibroblasts and keratinocytes, as well as receptors for hormones, neuropeptides, and neurotransmitters. This allows the skin to provide critical data to all organ systems, which is especially pertinent when the skin is challenged by an environmental stressor like the sun or physical and mental stress. Much more than just a physical barrier, the skin functions very much like the brain or the endocrine system by providing important information to the body.

These receptor sites allow the skin to receive messages via neurotransmitters, neuropeptides, hormones, and nerve impulses. This information provides the basis for what is known as the mind-body connection, which is much more than a New Age concept. Scientists have shown that there is a very real connection. The skin functions as an information superhighway that provides us with vital tools to understand and diagnose diseases of the skin as well as mental diseases and disorders. Just by stimulating the skin, you can actually change the chemistry in your brain. Conversely, anxiety attacks and depression will affect your skin. Stimulating the skin can activate the autonomic nervous system, specifically the rest-and-digest parasympathetic side, and enhance secretion of the Beauty Molecule and all of its benefits.

The receptors in the skin via the neuropeptides of the skin formed the basis of the topical and supplement form of the neuroceuticals that I developed and introduced more than two decades ago. One of the premier active ingredients in my patented Perricone formulations for cosmeceuticals, which I introduced in 1997, is dimethylaminoethanol (DMAE). DMAE's dual function in the skin and the brain makes it the ideal ingredient for neuroceuticals and neurocosmeceuticals. Like acetylcholine, neuroceuticals are major factors in creating and maintaining beautiful, radiant, and youthful-looking skin.

GLUTATHIONE, THE MASTER ANTIOXIDANT

Glutathione is a tripeptide, a molecule composed of three amino acids. It is the most abundant and important antioxidant protective system in our cells. I have written about glutathione many times over the years. As I wrote in my past book *Forever Young,* glutathione is critical in the cells' defense against inflammation-generating free radicals and oxidative stress. When cells are under severe oxidative stress, they produce glutathione as an antioxidant to resist the oxidative stress.

In addition to being a critical part of our antioxidant defense system, glutathione is an important detoxifying agent, which enables the body to eliminate toxins and poisons. This detoxification is critical in providing protection against chemicals that promote cell transformation or cell death. Glutathione also regulates and regenerates our immune cells. People with chronic illnesses such as AIDS, cancer, and autoimmune diseases generally have very low levels of glutathione.

Glutathione has another role in protecting enzyme proteins that inhibit collagen-digesting enzymes that cause damage to the skin, leading to wrinkles or scars from acne lesions.

It is almost impossible to overstate glutathione's importance as the body's primary antioxidant defense system. Required for the smooth functioning of all cells, glutathione is involved in protein synthesis, amino acid transport, and the recycling of other antioxidants like vitamin C, vitamin E, and CoQ10 to assist their function in protecting the cell.

Unfortunately, glutathione levels decrease as we age. But all is not lost.

GlyNAC TO THE RESCUE

During my research I discovered a remarkable study titled "Supplementing Glycine and N-Acetylcysteine (GlyNAC) in Older Adults Improves Glutathione Deficiency, Oxidative Stress, Mitochondrial Dysfunction, Inflammation, Physical Function, and Aging Hallmarks" in *The Journals of Gerontology, Series A, Biological Sciences and Medical Sciences*. This article is available to everyone on the National Library of Medicine's website at https://pubmed.ncbi.nlm.nih.gov/35975308/.

As glutathione levels decrease with age, we lose the vital protection this master antioxidant bestows. The unique combination of the two amino acids glycine and N-acetylcysteine, known as GlyNAC, provides a solution to this problem. The study found that after 16 weeks of supplementation with GlyNAC in older adults a wide variety of aging hallmarks improved or were corrected. These age-related problems include oxidative stress, lower glutathione levels, mitochondrial dysfunction, inflammation, endothelial dysfunction, insulin resistance, impaired physical function, increased waist circumference, and raised systolic blood pressure. The authors of this study concluded that by combining the benefits of glycine and NAC, GlyNAC is an effective nutritional supplement that improves and reverses multiple age-associated abnormalities to promote health in aging humans.

THE INCREDIBLE BENEFITS OF GlyNAC

There are many benefits to glycine:

- Prevents inflammation
- Increases production of glutathione
- Protects the heart
- Protects the liver
- Aids digestion
- Improves quality of sleep
- Assists in memory
- Helps boost mental performance
- Aids in joint repair by protecting collagen
- Helps alleviate joint pain
- Assists in joint mobility, and range of motion
- Increases collagen production in both skin and joints
- Helps build lean muscle mass
- Protects against muscle loss (sarcopenia)
- Aids in metabolic disorders
- Stabilizes blood sugar thereby lowering risk of type 2 diabetes
- Aids in production of human growth hormone
- Protects against ischemic stroke and seizures
- Helps in reducing allergic reactions

When we are older, we have about 25 percent of the glutathione we had when we were young. Supplementing with GlyNAC will restore glutathione to significantly higher levels—almost to the same levels of our youth, rejuvenating our organ systems on a subcellular level and repairing mitochondria in all organ systems, making it an indispensable addition to our healthful aging arsenal.

ALISON'S STORY

Alison is a respected journalist for a renowned beauty magazine. We have kept in touch over the years. Always on the hunt for exciting news, she often called just to catch up. Alison knows my dedication to staying abreast of the latest research—especially in the arcane area of cell biology. Our last phone call in early March was no exception.

As ever, Alison was eager for the latest news and wanted me to update her on what her readers needed to know. With her usual cut to the chase, she also wanted to know what she needed to look 10 years younger.

Although I always had important updates for restoring beauty and health, I was brimming over with exciting new breakthroughs on this particular call. I asked her if she had heard of GlyNAC. When Alison confirmed that this was the first she had heard if it, I spent the next 30 minutes bringing her up to date. I told her the tale of two simple amino acids and their near miraculous abilities to reverse a significant number of the signs of aging.

After a consultation with her primary care physician, Alison began a faithful regimen of taking 6 grams of glycine and 6 grams of NAC each morning on an empty stomach. The glycine bulk powder that she purchased on Amazon had a 3-gram scoop in the jar so she was able to use that. Because NAC has such an unpleasant taste, I recommended that she use the tablets instead of the powder, taking three tablets of 1000 mg daily. The dose for both the glycine and NAC was based on the clinical trials and her body weight of 122 pounds.

According to many studies, GlyNAC has been shown to repair a host of aging hallmarks present in older people, defects linked to oxidative stress and impaired mitochondrial function. These defects include inflammation, insulin resistance, and endothelial dysfunction, all of which increase our risk of coronary artery disease. Other areas of action target declining strength and cognition and the development of sarcopenia, age-related loss of muscle mass and gaining of body fat.

Although Alison was only in her mid- to late forties, she admitted that she often felt tired. When it came to her skin, she confessed that the bloom was off the rose.

One of the major culprits for both elevated oxidative stress and mito-chondrial dysfunction in older people is the deficiencies of the antioxidant tripeptide glutathione (GSH) and its precursor amino acids glycine and N-acetylcysteine, which may contribute to those problems. Researchers have dis-covered that supplementation with GlyNAC could significantly restore levels of glutathione. Believe me when I say this is a major breakthrough in treating aging and age-related diseases—from sagging, wrinkled skin to heart disease.

Under a brilliant blue sky and balmy temperatures, I made my way out to the Hamptons for a Fourth of July fundraiser. It had been more than four months since I had last seen or spoken to Alison. But there she was in a midriff-baring top paired with matching shorts—a vision in white and the center of much attention. Alison quickly broke away from her admirers to come over to say hello.

Alison was delighted to see me and confessed that she could not wait to share the results of her GlyNAC experience. She told me she had been a faithful adherent for more than four months, and the difference in how she looked and felt was nothing short of astounding. She was thrilled that she even got her waistline back.

I knew firsthand that improving body composition is one of the visible benefits of GlyNAC. I had seen my own muscle mass increase along with the loss of body fat. Observing the changes in Alison really brought it all home. She not only looked significantly younger, she also radiated a youthful vitality that cannot be faked.

I have always said that true beauty is radiant health, and there in front of me stood living proof. I knew that Alison's physical transformation was a powerful reflection of the mitochondrial repair taking place on a cellular level along with a major decrease in inflammation in all her organ systems.

As studies continue to mount, it appears that GlyNAC is introducing a transformative paradigm shift in aging and the entire field of geriatrics. By restoring youthful levels of glutathione, we can now reverse multiple aging hallmarks. In addition to offering protection from major disease, GlyNac helps to improve strength, exercise capacity, cognition, and body composi-tion. Good news indeed!

GETTING STARTED

I began using the pure powders of glycine and NAC (N-acetylcysteine) and recommending it to my patients rather than the GlyNAC capsules that combine the two. However, the NAC powder was unpalatable and difficult to stick with. So I recommend the tablets (not the capsules) that are available on Amazon. This supplement is recommended for healthy individuals, 18 years and older. According to *Medical News Today*, 600 mg to 1,200 mg is the most commonly recommended dosage of GlyNAC by medical practitioners. The study used larger amounts that should be under the supervision of your physician. Consult a healthcare professional prior to use if you are pregnant, nursing, taking medication, or have a medical condition. If you are taking blood pressure medication, be certain to check with your doctor before starting on this supplement, because it can lower your blood pressure too much.

NEUROPEPTIDES AND THE BRAIN-BEAUTY CONNECTION

DMAE became a cornerstone ingredient in a line of anti-aging skin treatments I developed decades ago, all thanks to an aha! moment during my residency, when I realized that what is therapeutic for the brain can be equally therapeutic and healing for the skin. DMAE is instrumental in increasing the production of acetylcholine, the Beauty Molecule, the heart and soul of this book. Throughout this period of working with DMAE, I continued to be fascinated by the brain-beauty connection. I began my research into this connection more than 30 years ago. That research laid the foundation for my discovery of the Beauty Molecule, acetylcholine. I was intrigued by the fact that the fine tuning of neurotransmission was produced by tiny strings of amino acids known as neuropeptides.

When I started to study neuropeptides, my first step was to discover if there were receptors in the skin for these peptides. I felt strongly that there had to be because the skin and the brain are directly connected from the embryonic state. The answer was a resounding yes, there *were* receptors in the skin for the neuropeptides. In creating topical formulations, I chose the neuropeptides that had anti-inflammatory activity and made the first products with the penetration enhancers. After applying the new formulations to skin, I was impressed by the results. The powerful anti-inflammatory properties the neuropeptides exhibited showed significant reparative activity on skin. I wasted no time in applying for the patents necessary to protect this exciting new technology, and they were issued soon after my application.

Synthesizing the neuropeptides was a hugely expensive process. The cost ranged anywhere from $30,000 to $50,000 per kilo, and I was concerned that this cost would demand a price that would be prohibitive to customers. When the president of a prestigious department store asked me if I had anything new in the pipeline, I shared my concern. I explained that I was enthusiastic about the neuropeptide products but was worried about the pricing. He told me that the store had been selling some very expensive products, and those were not functioning anywhere near the level of mine. He encouraged me to go ahead and create the products for retail. Even though the products would be costly, he was confident that the price would not be an issue with his customers. He was right. The neuropeptide line generated tremendous brand loyalty and became a runaway success for many years. When the line of neuropeptide products was so well received, I was inspired to continue and expand my research in this field.

MITOCHONDRIAL-DERIVED PEPTIDES

I have been focusing on recent peptide discoveries, including peptides known as mitochondrial-derived peptides. Mitochondrial-derived peptides are small peptides expressed by the mitochondrial genome (DNA). Scientists thought until recently that the mitochondrial DNA was just directing the building plans for the mitochondria itself. We now know that the genome is also responsible for creating mitochondrial-derived peptides that circulate and have benefit throughout the entire body. Mitochondrial-derived peptides preserve mitochondrial functions, protect all organ systems, and protect stressed cells. Scientists agree that elevating the levels of these protective mitochondrial peptides could bring health and longevity benefits above physiologic production. And like the Ashkenazi Jews, many of whom live to 100 years or more, perhaps extend our lifespan beyond 100 years.

Three variations of the mitochondrial-derived peptides have been identified: humanin, MOTS-c, and a group designated SHLP1–6. Much of the major work on mitochondrial derived peptides has been done by Dr. Pinchas Cohen, professor of gerontology, medicine, and biological sciences at UC Davis and dean of the USC Leonard Davis School of Gerontology. Dr. Cohen discovered and named the peptide humanin, which has a powerful protective activity against the aging process. Humanin is a 24-amino acid peptide encoded from the mt-16S-rRNA.

These peptides have metabolic and anti-aging benefits. Mitochondrial-derived peptides are protective of the brain and could be the key to preventing or reversing cognitive decline in the future. These mitochondrial-derived peptides can change metabolism in a healthful way, increase stamina and muscle mass, and protect the heart, brain, liver, and kidneys. Because these peptides are created in the mitochondrial DNA and are physiologically active, they are totally benign substances.

Harking back to the brain-beauty connection, I was intrigued by the concept of topically applying the mitochondrial-derived peptides. Knowing that aging begins in the mitochondria, I was fascinated by the idea that such a peptide coming from the mitochondria itself could hold the key to aging. These peptides activate the sirtuins, proteins with anti-aging activity. They provide powerful neuroprotection that maintains and extends brain health and good cognitive function.

The problem with these peptides is that they have to be administered by injection. If we took the peptides orally, they would be broken up by our digestive system, losing their efficacy. Even when injected, the life of peptides is short, with some as low as 30 minutes. I turned to my transdermal biotechnology company and looked for a formula that could deliver the peptide while stabilizing and preserving the activity. By putting the peptides into a transdermal cream, a safe and nontoxic delivery system, much greater benefits were derived than from the injection of these peptides. The transdermal liquid crystal carrier prevents enzymes that would degrade the structure, compromising their efficacy. Much to our delight, we found that humanin, the mitochondrial-derived protein, was effective in this transdermal delivery system and increased its biological activity from a mere 30 minutes to hours. Now we were able to deliver these extraordinary therapeutic effects with much greater efficacy than by injection.

Humanin is a remarkable discovery. The scientists doing the research looked at a large group of Ashkenazi Jews, who are noted for longevity. The scientists chose this group because a large percentage of these people lived to 100 years or more. These centenarians have much higher levels of humanin in their bodies than the general population. The scientists then looked at the children of these centenarians and found that they too had much higher levels of humanin than age-matched control subjects. Further linking humanin to health span, one of the studies observed that humanin levels are decreased in human diseases such as Alzheimer's disease, mitochondrial encephalopathy, lactic acidosis, and stroke-like episodes.

Humanin is benign and has great ability to maintain cellular health. It has very powerful anti-inflammatory activity in the central nervous system. Maintaining healthy brain function as we age is central to successful aging. We can apply humanin to the skin in transdermal form and receive its therapeutic benefits.

I am very excited about our research studying the mitochondrial-derived peptides and the possibility of administering them transdermally. This efficient delivery system makes these peptides more available and more effective.

For those of us trying to preserve both our lifespan and health span, these peptides offer great benefit when applied topically with the right penetration enhancers. They will not only increase the youthful appearance of skin, but also protect cells against various diseases, including diabetes mellitus and cardiovascular and neurodegenerative diseases. Humanin exerts pro-apoptotic activity of TNF-alpha in cancer, which also makes it a novel therapeutic agent. TNF-alpha, a micropeptide encoded in the mitochondrial genome, protects cells from diverse pathological conditions, including neural and skeletal diseases.

THE PEPTIDE WEIGHT LOSS
BREAKTHROUGH

While it may have taken mainstream science more than two decades to catch up to my original teachings, the old adage "better late than never" again rings true. I find it both satisfying and gratifying to see my work validated—not because I needed other researchers to substantiate or attest to my findings. Instead, I am delighted to see them play catch-up and finally address the link between aging, metabolism, and inflammation.

I knew that inflammation was always the origin and the final common pathway in degenerative diseases, especially those linked to aging. Although this universal theory of inflammation was not well accepted (I am being polite here as the truth is this theory was openly ridiculed), progress in addressing this inflammation is finally taking center stage.

Let's start with twin scourges of today's Western society—diabetes and obesity. Major pharmaceutical companies have now been developing new treatments for type 2 diabetes and obesity. They are looking at specific hormones released by the small intestine called incretins. Incretins are gut-derived peptide hormones that are rapidly secreted in response to a meal. The two main incretins in humans are glucose-dependent insulinotropic polypeptide (GIP) and glucagon-like peptide-1 (GLP-1). They stimulate pancreatic beta cells postprandially (after eating), to secrete insulin.

Simply put, these incretins are gut peptides that are released by the small intestine after eating to cause an insulin response or to secrete insulin to maintain normal blood sugar.

Scientists at the pharmaceutical companies have created a molecule that simulates the activity of these incretins, GIP and GLP-1, the goal being to increase their half-life, as it only lasts for about 8 to 10 minutes in the bloodstream. GLP-1 has a variety of functions, including inhibition of glucagon secretion, suppression of appetite, and slowing of gastric emptying, helping us to feel satiated longer. All of which are important in prevention of overeating. But that is not all. Due to these effects, incretins and incretin-mimetic drugs are commonly used to treat insulin resistance and type 2 diabetes. One distinct advantage of this class of drug is the lack of weight gain frequently associated with type 2 diabetes medications, and in fact some patients lose weight. Because of this they are increasing in popularity as an important adjunct in weight control programs. Disadvantages include an increased risk of hypoglycemia.

Unfortunately, both GIP and GLP-1 are rapidly degraded after their secretion by a major enzyme known as dipeptidyl peptidase 4 (DPP-4), resulting in their inactivation.

To prevent this breakdown and thereby increase the length of time that these incretins would be active, the scientists altered the sequence of amino acids and added a fatty acid chain that results in circulating levels of these hormones. Instead of mere minutes, these molecules can now mimic the natural hormone for days. They can now attach to and activate the same receptor sites more effectively than the native hormones. This results in remarkable responses in that there is decreased appetite, normalization of metabolism, and an increase in the efficiency of energy production. When such a new molecule is designed and attaches to the receptor sites, it is known as an agonist.

In the patients now being treated with these pharmaceuticals, we are seeing remarkable weight loss and normalization of blood sugar, helping to eradicate type 2 diabetes and decrease body fat.

COMING FULL CIRCLE

What I find particularly interesting and satisfying about these developments is the ability of these synthetic hormones to mimic the effects of the anti-inflammatory diet that I designed decades ago. This unequivocally proves the fundamental, intrinsic link connecting metabolism to inflammation.

While these pharmaceuticals were developed for control of diabetes and obesity, they are impacting all organ systems with positive effects, in the same manner as my anti-inflammatory diet. Reducing inflammation on a systemic level can now be achieving with an injection. But the news gets even better.

Due to the powerful anti-inflammatory effects, I predict that the custom-made peptide will be used across a broad spectrum of debilitating diseases and conditions. This will include neural protection, in both the prevention and perhaps treatment of Alzheimer's disease as well as Parkinson's disease. They may also be vital in cardiac health, repairing the heart muscle and preventing atherosclerosis through their anti-inflammatory activity. Their ability to rejuvenate mitochondria in all cells in our body will provide us with protection for all major organ systems, including healthier liver and kidney function, stronger muscle tissue, better bone density, arthritis treatment and prevention, younger and more resilient skin, enhanced brain function, and increased immune function. In short, these anti-inflammatory properties will provide comprehensive, far-ranging, and far-reaching benefits. And of course intimately involved in this cascade of health and beauty benefits is acetylcholine, the beauty molecule, activating the autonomic nervous system, bringing balance to all organ systems offering powerful anti-inflammatory effects. In short, maximum health and beauty benefits with minimal side effects This is what we were achieving with the anti-inflammatory diet, and it now appears that this new peptide can offer equally powerful anti-inflammatory effects.

Current research focuses on several different pharmaceuticals. I have personally observed patients using tirzepatide, a weekly treatment designed for obesity. Just as only 3 days on the anti-inflammatory diet will deliver visible results, such as changes in skin radiance, tone, and a decrease in visible wrinkles, these patients not only lost weight, they looked markedly younger in a very short period of time.

The really good news is that the peptide that forms the basis of these pharmaceuticals can be put into a transdermal solution and applied topically. Now we can avoid injections as well as avoid having to take a prescription drug. An extremely low percentage of this peptide can be used to cosmetically rejuvenate skin without systemic effects. This provides us with a physiological alternative in managing inflammation—without side effects. As we know, physiological means to work *with* the body, unlike pharmaceuticals. It is related to the branch of biology that deals with the normal functions of living organisms and their parts. So not only effective, but natural and compatible with our bodies.

Based on the Beauty Molecule, we now have another complementary and highly effective therapy to add to our armamentarium to control inflammation.

Understanding the role of peptides and neuropeptides is not just limited to our health and our lifespan—but is vital to our very existence! The neuropeptides play many roles in our physical bodies as well as influencing our emotional, spiritual, mental, and psychological health. In fact, it is not a stretch to learn that neuropeptides also have important influence on our choices of a mate. When we understand the mysteries of nature and how the survival of a species depends upon these, the subtle messaging from parts of our brain and other organ systems, it opens up new doors of perception—as we will discover in the upcoming chapter.

8

NEUROPEPTIDES AND THE LAWS OF ATTRACTION

LONG CONSIDERED A MYSTERY OF the ages, physical attraction has often defied explanation. What is that certain something that makes us choose one partner over another? In nature, the answer appears to lie in something known as pheromones. But what are they exactly and are they really a contributing factor in that elusive but powerful magnetism we feel towards someone—a magnetism that can even override common sense?

UNDERSTANDING PHEROMONES

A pheromone is defined in zoology as a chemical substance produced and released into the environment by an animal, especially a mammal or an insect, that affects the behavior or physiology of others of its species. Though this definition may seem dry, the reality is anything but. Discussing pheromones involves the intriguing science behind the wealth of human emotions.

The human limbic system, varying little from that of more primitive animals, is where the inherent responses required for survival of a species are believed to originate. Often thought of as a minibrain, our limbic system largely controls our behavior and our emotions. The most ancient and primitive part of the brain, the limbic system is at the core of our emotions. Learning and memory are also within the range of its function.

Our sense of smell, via our olfactory receptors, has a direct impact on the body and the emotions. Relating the association of a smell with an emotional reaction occurs because our olfactory receptors are directly connected to the limbic system. There are two sets of receptor cells in the nose. In addition to the main set, which detects general odors, we have receptors for human axillary secretions like pheromones.

Pheromones are in the axillary sweat found on the surface of the skin in the armpits. This sweat interacts with bacteria, creating pheromones that activate those receptors in the human nose, triggering a wide range of human emotions. Covering the entire emotional gamut, these emotions range from love to hate and from happiness to misery. Although different from those found in the animal and insect worlds, these emotions have a profound effect on human physiology and behavior. The physical effect can be seen in the coordination of the menstrual cycles of women who live in close proximity, the bonding of the child with the mother through release of oxytocin during breastfeeding, and the cooperation and bonding shown when groups of people do physical work together. Perceiving these axillary pheromones activates the parasympathetic nervous system, the rest-and-digest portion of the autonomic nervous system.

THE NEUROPEPTIDE CONNECTION

Some pheromones are neuropeptides, which are peptides composed of short chains of amino acids released by neurons in the brain that act as intercellular messengers. Some neuropeptides function as neurotransmitters and others as hormones. In addition to the major neurotransmitters, including dopamine, norepinephrine, and serotonin, pheromones are extremely important in controlling our moods and our brain. Neurotransmitters do a fine-tuning, while neuropeptides, including the pheromones, do an even finer tuning. The rates at which our brain, skin, and organ systems age are controlled by the vast intracellular network that makes up the endocrine and nervous systems.

First discovered in insects in 1959, pheromones are used to attract members of the opposite sex, to mark trails and territory, and as warnings. The chemical messages sent by the pheromones are a powerful form of communication between members of the same animal and insect species, unlike hormones, which act on an individual.

THE LAWS OF ATTRACTION

Our pheromones give off a certain odor based on the immune signature of our cells. This immune signature is known as the major histocompatibility complex (MHC). The MHC is a group of genes that controls aspects of the immune response. Studies have found that mice nest with other mice that have genes compatible with their own MHC, because they feel safe with these mice. But there is a dramatic change when these mice reach puberty. They then look for mates whose genes are different from their own, to ensure a more diverse gene pool.

"Pheromones and Their Effect on Women's Mood and Sexuality" is a fascinating study published in *Facts, Views & Vision in ObGyn* (https://www.ncbi.nlm.nih.gov/pmc/articles/PMC3987372/). This study shows that pheromones may be present in all bodily secretions, but most attention has been geared toward axillary or armpit sweat, which contains the odorous 16-androstenes. Androstenedione, a steroidal hormone produced in male and female gonads as well as in the adrenal glands, is known for its role in the production of estrogen and testosterone. Androstenedione is present at much higher concentrations in male sweat and can be detected by women, albeit with wide variation in sensitivity. This study applied a pharmacological dose of androstenedione to the upper lip of women, resulting in improved mood and heightened focus. A positive mood is known to facilitate women's sexual response, and increased focus improves sexual satisfaction, desire, and arousal. The study concluded that some data indicate that 16-androstene pheromones, in particular androstenedione, play a beneficial role in women's mood, focus, and sexual response, and perhaps in mate selection.

As interest in pheromones intensified, ABC News conducted an informal test on human synthetic hormones on a once-popular news magazine show, 20/20. The producers decided to test whether pheromones had any effect on the opposite sex. The question was: Could pheromones help people find romance?

To find the answer, the show sent sets of male and female twins in their twenties to a speed dating event and provided each set with a scent. One twin in each set received a scent containing commercially available pheromones. The other twin had a scent without the pheromone. No one knew who had which scent. As ABC reported: "The female twins, Bridget and Sarah, were introduced to us through twinsworld.com. They said they would be convinced the pheromones worked if one of them was approached by more men at the speed-dating event."

They went on 10 dates, each lasting 5 minutes. The daters then filled out forms stating which of the people they would like to see again.

At the end of the night the results were tallied. Nine men wanted to see Sarah again and 5 men wanted to see Bridget again. As for the guys, 10 women were interested in Dave and only 6 women were interested in Paul.

Sarah and Dave were wearing the pheromones.

Although anecdotal and by no means scientific, it is a fascinating story. In pheromone studies, the pheromone solutions are often applied to the skin of study participants. Given that they affect physical parameters, including the autonomic nervous system, pheromones are proving to be a viable relationship enhancement strategy.

INTRODUCING THE GROUNDBREAKING AROMATIC NEURO-ENHANCER

Understanding pheromones and their potential impact is an intriguing premise. This knowledge has led me to research and develop an advanced aromatic neuro-enhancer. This unique proprietary blend of pheromones and neuropeptides represents a breakthrough as a new and exciting adjunct to enhancing personal and social relationships.

As I continued my research into perfecting and fine-tuning this formula, I learned even more. This aromatic neuro-enhancer is not just a relationship enhancer—as desirable and necessary as that is—it is also a powerful anti-aging aromatic, which can effectively manage our stress levels. Doing so is important, because stress weakens the immune system and makes the body more susceptible to aging and disease. Counteracting the negative by-products of stress, this new formula increases our sense of well-being. I believe it represents the next generation of rejuvenating treatment serums. It is not a traditional anti-aging serum applied to the skin for cosmetic results, but instead an innovative, therapeutic, and rejuvenating treatment for the brain. An added benefit: a delicate and delightful hint of fragrance.

Neurotransmitters play a crucial role in sending signals between nerve cells in the brain. By enhancing neurotransmitter activity, neuroceuticals are designed to facilitate faster and more effective communication, resulting in improved skin health and beauty. This aromatic neuro-enhancer captures the very essence of what the term "neuroceuticals" represents. It is the purest and most concentrated essence of the brain-beauty synergy.

What It Is

This formula is the first aromatic to combine pheromones with the advanced technology of the messenger neuropeptides that fine-tune brain chemistry. As you have learned, pheromones are the chemical messengers that communicate between individuals of all types and genders and are Nature's secret code designed to elicit behavioral or neuroendocrine responses.

Neuropeptides enhance the efficacy of human pheromones. The synergistic combination of these two messenger systems is incorporated in this proprietary formula, which offers unique benefits that exceed the effects of the ingredients when used individually.

Why It Works

Studies indicate there are multiple benefits in stimulating the olfactory nerves responsible for our sense of smell. Enhancing olfactory cells boosts the effects of odors and pheromones. We call this olfactory enrichment, which results in cognitive resilience. A recent study indicated that olfactory enrichment improves memory, perception, discernment, and awareness. Another study examining older patients with dementia found that olfactory enrichment enhanced memory, focus, and word finding. Science has discovered a 250 percent improvement in cognitive skills resulting from olfactory enrichment. This means the nerves in the brain form new synapses that increase cognitive resilience.

What It Does

The two sets of the receptor sites in the nose function in this manner. The main set detects general odors, and the other set responds to the axillary pheromones, which are separate from the activation of the sense of smell. Scientists have begun to recognize that pheromones directly activate a host of human emotions. This fact alone makes it an indispensable tool for the development of any and all interpersonal relationships and interactions.

When pheromones are perceived by the brain, they stimulate the release of neuropeptides, and they can then adhere to the receptor sites. This allows them to carry their various messages to different parts of the brain, affecting areas related to our sense of well-being, enhanced thinking, and emotional attraction. These messages also serve to activate the parasympathetic nervous system. As you have learned, increasing the activation of the rest-and-digest parasympathetic nervous systems increases vagal tone. When increased, vagal tone activates the Beauty Molecule, acetylcholine, which repairs mitochondria and activates AMPK.

THE BENEFICIAL EFFECTS PRODUCED BY AROMATIC NEURO-ENHANCEMENT

The right combination of neuropeptides and pheromones can provide many positive effects, including:

PHYSIOLOGICAL AND PSYCHOLOGICAL INTRAPERSONAL EFFECTS

- Increasing sense of well-being
- Exerting anti-inflammatory activity in the brain
- Elevating mood
- Helping lift depression that results from inflammation
- Enhancing memory and mental clarity
- Increasing self-confidence
- Sharpening problem-solving skills
- Improving cerebral blood flow
- Decreasing confusion
- Reducing levels of the stress hormones cortisol and adrenaline with the activation of the parasympathetic nervous system

INTERPERSONAL EFFECTS

- Increasing cooperation in group settings

OTHER TRANSDERMAL NEUROPEPTIDES

The peptide thyrotropin-releasing hormone (TRH) was brought to my attention by Dr. Walter Pierpaoli, who greatly expanded our knowledge of this peptide. Dr. Pierpaoli claimed that TRH is a misnomer, because this amazing peptide has many other activities beyond the thyroid. Dr. Pierpaoli's study, "Aging-Reversing Properties of Thyrotropin-Releasing

Hormone," was published in *Current Aging Science* (https://pubmed.ncbi .nlm.nih.gov/23895526). His study examined the effects of TRH on organs, tissues, and aging-related metabolic and hormonal markers. These experiments with TRH supplementation show the delaying and even rejuvenating effects of this neuropeptide.

The broad spectrum of TRH activities suggest that TRH has a fundamental role in the regulation of metabolic and hormonal functions. TRH is a powerful anti-aging agent with a number of positive effects, including anti-inflammatory activity and normalization of metabolic functions.

In addition to its physical effects, TRH also exerts significant mental and mood-influencing properties, exhibiting antidepressant activity and decreased suicidal ideation. The US Army began studying this aspect of TRH to help prevent suicide in returning soldiers. The studies have not proved successful because TRH does not traverse the blood-brain barrier. They have tried nasal sprays, as well as designing a study in which they placed TRH on swabs and inserted them into the nose, leaving them there for several minutes in an attempt to get the TRH into the brain.

The transdermal system I have developed utilizes a liquid crystal able to carry TRH through the skin into the bloodstream. Currently TRH is an effective peptide in this carrier thanks to its powerful anti-aging, metabolic-normalizing, and anti-inflammatory properties.

Dr. Pierpaoli's research in animals and humans indicates that TRH has a role in the regulation of metabolic and hormonal functions. Other studies show that people with higher levels of TRH in the brain have lower risk of cognitive decline. This peptide is proven to be a powerful and indispensable support for beauty, health, and longevity.

NEUROPEPTIDE Y

Neuropeptide Y (NPY), a 36-amino-acid peptide neurotransmitter, is the most powerful neuropeptide for promoting positive energy balance. This neuropeptide has various activities in the body, specifically in the brain and the peripheral nervous system. Produced in the brain, NPY functions to increase resilience in stressful and anxiety-producing situations by enhancing homeostasis, increasing stability and balance in major organ systems, and increasing neurogenesis, forming new neurons in the brain.

Studies from the military on neuropeptide Y and post-traumatic stress disorder (PTSD) have shown that soldiers with higher levels of neuropeptide Y in the brain have reduced incidence of PTSD, which results in greater resilience in stressful situations such as combat. Neuropeptide Y has anxiolytic or anti-anxiety effects, making it an effective treatment in stress-related environments. NPY's ability to decrease levels of stress and anxiety helps to prevent substance abuse, depression, suicide, and other serious mental disorders. Another side effect of NPY is decreased alcohol consumption, because NYP increases dopamine, which enhances feelings of well-being and stabilizes mood.

The transdermal system is the only effective method of administrating NPY. This method ensures that the neuropeptide will not be broken down by enzymes, and allows it passage through the blood-brain barrier. The administration of NPY with my patented transdermal formulation provides a workable solution to a major problem. Being able to increase levels of neuropeptide Y is an important anti-aging, anti-inflammatory addition to viable health and longevity strategies.

OXYTOCIN

Oxytocin (oxy or OT), a peptide hormone and neuropeptide, is normally produced in the hypothalamus and released into the bloodstream by the pituitary gland. In addition to stimulating uterine contractions in childbirth and lactation after childbirth, this natural hormone affects the male and female reproductive systems and aspects of human behavior. Released during lovemaking, OT is often referred to as the "love drug" or "love hormone." Oxytocin is instrumental in human bonding. Breastfeeding mothers create a bond with their infants through the secretion of this neuropeptide. The hormone is also released during orgasm.

Oxytocin can help to form bonding during group meetings and enhance synergy and cooperation; I use oxytocin transdermally prior to meetings. In fact, I started a small club in which a group of us get together and use oxytocin transdermally prior to meetings to enhance synergy and cooperation. We call it the James Bonding Club. Communication is greatly enhanced and we really have a great time. The prosocial neuropeptide oxytocin has been shown to enhance social functioning and bonding in both healthy and clinical populations, and may have the ability to facilitate unit cohesion and teamwork in military settings, ultimately helping to prevent and treat the psychological trauma experienced by veterans.

A TRUE STORY

One person asked me for some topical oxytocin in hopes of creating a deeper relationship with someone she was interested in. I agreed but advised that she tell him she was using a lotion designed to form bonds with those she was interacting with.

Fast-forward a month and a half. I received a frantic call from her telling me that the man in question was driving her nuts. He wouldn't leave her alone.

I asked if she had used the transdermal. She answered that she had. When I asked if she had told him, she confessed that she hadn't.

"Well, I don't know how we put that particular genie back in the bottle—you will just have to tell him face-to-face that you are not interested in pursuing a romantic relationship," I replied, hoping that would be enough to put a damper on his ardor. I chuckled, thinking this was a classic case of "be careful what you wish for."

Oxytocin, dopamine, and serotonin are often referred to as our "happy hormones." When you are attracted to another person, your brain releases dopamine, your serotonin levels increase, and oxytocin is produced. This causes you to feel a surge of positive emotion.

Oxytocin decreases stress while enhancing interpersonal relationships, making it another important addition to our anti-aging and increased-well-being strategies.

PART 2

STRATEGIES TO PROMOTE AND SUPPORT THE BEAUTY MOLECULE

9

THE PERRICONE
DAILY ROUTINE

YOU MAY BE WONDERING HOW to put the science and information you have read in part 1 to use in your everyday life. The many benefits of an anti-inflammatory lifestyle are certainly motivating. In this part of the book, I focus on strategies that will stimulate production of the Beauty Molecule, acetylcholine, and keep you young on a cellular level. Each chapter in part 2 explains how to use the strategies. You will learn how to regulate your circadian rhythm, how to add more movement and exercise into your life without having to work out in a gym for hours at a time, and how to fight inflammation with deep breathing and a variety of meditation techniques. You have probably heard about intermittent fasting and might wonder if you have the stamina to try it. The chapter covering this subject includes several fasting options that allow you to ease your way into the practice. The last chapter covers a strategy that is near and dear to my heart: as a dermatologist, I have a lot to say about topicals that will make you radiant.

After many years of study and research, trial and error, I believe the routine I now follow significantly contributes to my overall health and well-being. People often ask me what they can do to optimize their mental and physical fitness, which is why I am sharing my own personal program, one that I follow faithfully every day. This routine is tailored for me and my needs. As you become acquainted with the various strategies, you will be able to set up a regimen that works with the shape of your day and the time that you have. Many of you will have issues that you want to address, such as reducing stress, breaking out of a sedentary lifestyle, enhancing your energy, falling asleep more easily, or resisting food cravings. The chapters that follow are designed to give you methods of doing something positive to fight inflammation and to achieve calmness, good health, restored energy, and longevity, and supple, glowing skin.

As I describe my routine, I will reiterate a variety of biological reasons these actions work. Although the science may be covered elsewhere in this book, I am repeating myself because I am demonstrating the strategies "in action" to explain why I incorporate them in my daily regimen. Sometimes practical application helps us to understand the big picture, which is increased production of the Beauty Molecule, acetylcholine, for enhanced mental and physical well-being.

THE PERRICONE DAILY ROUTINE

On awakening in the morning, the first thing I do is to move to the brightest room in the house or, weather permitting, step outside dressed in the appropriate clothing for the season. My goal is to get the light from the sun into my eyes. Whether it is sunny or overcast, sunlight is the key to setting circadian rhythm, which I elaborate on in the next chapter. Your circadian rhythm controls your metabolism along with many other body functions. Controlled by the hypothalamus, the circadian rhythm also regulates the hormones of the endocrine system, the "master clock," and the sleep/wake cycle. By receiving bright, natural light directly into my eyes, I am setting the circadian rhythm for the day.

By getting the optimal light from the sun—even on an overcast, gray day, which takes a bit longer—I am setting my master clock and increasing my overall alertness. I like to linger in the morning light to get as much infrared exposure from the sun as possible for its therapeutic benefit.

When the eyes see the morning light, signals are sent to the hypothalamus. The body immediately stops producing melatonin, an extremely important antioxidant crucial for the production of the master antioxidant glutathione. When we sleep, melatonin is released by the pineal gland in the brain. The melatonin then circulates in our bloodstream and is taken up by the cells. The melatonin enters the mitochondria to protect them from free radical damage.

As important as it is to get exposure to the bright morning light to stop melatonin production and set our master clock, it is just as important to avoid light exposure at night, when we still need to protect our eyes from bright lights. Computer screens, cell phones, and television, for example, all generate blue light. Blue light turns off production of melatonin and triggers alertness. When I work on my computer at night, I wear glasses called "blue blockers," which prevent the blue light frequency from disrupting my circadian rhythm.

The sleep/wake cycle is profoundly involved in regulating our metabolism, which includes regulating blood sugar, blood fats, and cholesterol. When your circadian rhythm is disturbed, your metabolism is also disturbed. I have to emphasize how important it is to keep our metabolism regulated. If not, a variety of health problems, including cardiovascular disease, neurological decline, and even cancer, might develop.

The next step of my regimen is to perform a series of calisthenic exercises for about 15 to 20 minutes. Weather permitting, I exercise outside in the fresh air. The calisthenics I do in the early morning light give me time in the sun with low-ultraviolet rays and high levels of infrared light. Moving releases acetylcholine to the muscles to stimulate contractions. Then upregulation of the master metabolic regulator AMPK occurs, further normalizing my metabolism.

I do weight resistance training three times per week. Resistance training does not have to involve heavy weights or barbells. I use light weights and high repetitions to perform a variety of exercises during my 30-to-40-minute workout. On the days not devoted to weight training, I focus on stretching exercises for 15 minutes.

THE BIOLOGY OF EXERCISE

Resistance training and exercise activates many of the pathways discussed in earlier chapters. Exercise activates AMPK and affects the mTOR pathways, which lead to metabolic repair and adaptations that optimize our cellular metabolism.

Acetylcholine, the Beauty Molecule, has the power to increase production of these master switches, which enhance production of energy, improve mitochondrial function, and promote muscle mass by increasing protein synthesis.

Activation of mTOR promotes the growth of muscles. Frailty is a major risk factor as we age because it is a significant risk factor for death. By doing resistance exercises, you not only normalize metabolism, but also increase muscle mass, the key factor in preventing frailty. As we activate mTOR, muscle growth and repair and critical changes in metabolism begin. Performing exercises with light weights and high repetitions produces chemicals in the muscles. Lactate is one of them. Having positive effects on our metabolism, lactate can reduce appetite and at the same time increase production of the Beauty Molecule, acetylcholine.

Once lactic acid is produced in the muscles as a by-product of muscle contraction or movement, it teams up with an amino acid called phenylalanine. This lactate/phenylalanine molecule, known as Lac-Phe, is currently being studied for its neuroprotective properties and its ability to normalize metabolism. These properties have inspired me to produce a transdermal form of lactate and phenylalanine, which can be applied to the skin to provide neurological benefits, appetite suppression, and metabolism normalization.

BIOLOGICAL BENEFITS OF EXERCISE

Exercise activates a number of pathways. To summarize the effects:

AMPK

Resistance training, which involves muscle contraction, activates AMPK.

- AMPK acts as a sensor in our in our muscles, communicating that the cell is low on energy
- AMPK sets off metabolic responses that lower blood sugar, increase fat burning, preserve muscle mass, optimize cellular metabolism, and, most important, improve the function of our mitochondria

mTOR

Resistance training also stimulates mTOR, which:

- Regulates protein synthesis, cell growth, and muscle growth
- Acts as a nutrient energy center in the cell, particularly in the skeletal muscles
- Enhances protein synthesis to increase muscle mass
- Helps repair and build muscle tissue
- Contributes to metabolic repair by supporting anabolic cellular processes

LAC-PHE

- Lactate is produced as part of anaerobic metabolism in the muscle cells, which involves making energy without oxygen
- Lactate can then be absorbed by other cells, including in the brain, where it serves as an alternative energy source
- Lac-Phe normalizes metabolism and has neuroprotective properties

RESTORING YOUTHFUL CONTOURS

Exercising the body is not the only exercise that is important. As a dermatologist with a great interest in beauty, I was fascinated to learn about myofunctional therapy, a method said to restore youthful contours, muscle, and bone of the face without invasive surgery or fillers.

I first became aware of myofunctional therapy because I was experiencing a sleep disorder. Recent research had shown that myofunctional therapy can reduce the symptoms of sleep-disordered breathing such as snoring and ameliorate mild to moderate obstructive sleep apnea.

I was eager to learn more about this therapy after I met Marc Moeller, who was a fellow student and colleague of mine at the Yale School of Public Health. He introduced me to his mother, Joy Moeller, who has been a myofunctional therapist in private practice since 1980. She graduated from the Institute of Myofunctional Therapy in Coral Gables, Florida, and had an extensive internship in orofacial myology.

It was no surprise to me to learn that when functioning and used properly, the muscles of the tongue, throat, and face can reduce obstruction to the airway. This approach made a lot of sense to me, because it would help the body to heal naturally.

As I delved deeper into the science behind this therapy, I learned that orofacial myofunctional disorders (OMDs) are disorders of the muscles and functions of the face and mouth. OMDs may directly and/or indirectly affect breastfeeding, facial skeletal growth and development, chewing, swallowing, speech, occlusion, temporomandibular joint movement, oral hygiene, stability of orthodontic treatment, facial aesthetics, and more. I was already well on my way to curing my sleep/breathing problem with this therapy. The idea of the therapy's ability to alter facial aesthetics held great appeal. As we age, we begin to experience the loss of anatomic position of the face. Facial muscles get weaker over time. The loss of muscle tone, and thinning skin, can give the face a loose, sagging appearance. The jawline loses its contour, and our profile becomes less defined. Discovering a therapy that could improve facial muscle tone was exciting.

I was delighted when my course with Joy Moeller offered so much more than a cure to my sleep and breathing problem. The course consisted of a series of exercises of the tongue and mouth that slowly escalated in duration and repetition, with an expanded repertoire. As time passed, I noticed several positive changes in my appearance along with restored functional breathing.

When I read the literature on myofunctional therapy, I learned that there are reports of changes in bone structure due to the flexibility of the sutures, joints between the bones of the skull that hold them tightly together with fibrous tissue and allow flexibility and movement. The combination of movement and isotonic exercises has a dramatic and continued effect on appearance, first seen in weeks, with greater changes in months. Myofunctional therapy is effective for working facial muscles, restoring anatomic position and youthful contours, and restoring the bone and muscle structure of the face, throat, and neck area. If you want to learn more about the therapy, you will find helpful information at

- Joy Moeller's website (https://joymoeller.com)
- The Academy of Orofacial Myofunctional Therapy (https://aomtinfo.org)

I have had noticeable results, which is why I am telling you about the therapy.

BEAUTY FROM THE INSIDE OUT

My philosophy has always been "beauty from the inside out," accomplished by not only the anti-inflammatory diet, but also by taking supplements that have anti-inflammatory action. These include alpha-lipoic acid, vitamin C ester, DMAE, and the polyphenols that are found in olive oil, such as hydroxytyrosol, as well as peptides and neuropeptides. All of these substances work positively on the metabolic switch AMPK and at the same time upregulate the anti-aging proteins known as sirtuins, which are involved in regulating cellular processes, including the aging and death of cells and their resistance to stress.

I take supplements with hydrogen water because hydrogen water enhances the uptake of these nutrients. The hydrogen water has its own high level of anti-inflammatory effects and has been found to enhance the antioxidant capabilities of vitamins like C and E. Hydrogen water is called the intelligent antioxidant because it selectively neutralizes only highly toxic free radicals like the hydroxyl radical. Taking large amounts of antioxidants, which are not selective in the way hydrogen is, can result in reductive stress, the counterpart of oxidative stress. With reductive stress, the electron acceptors are reduced.

Many of the supplements I take have been part of my daily routine for years. Since my past book, I have added supplements based on what I learned about the on/off switches in our cells that affect metabolism and the anti-inflammatory response.

Nutritional supplements can enhance your efforts to bring your body back into a healthy balance that will boost your energy and turn back the clock. I have studied available supplements to pinpoint those that offer powerful protection from the often devastating effects of inflammation. Based on current research, my recommendations also reflect the results I have seen in my patients and myself.

I will focus on supplements that are fat metabolizers, energy boosters, antioxidants, anti-inflammatory, anti-aging and, most important, Beauty Molecule (acetylcholine) inducing. Though some of these supplements may not be familiar, they are all readily available.

You may not necessarily have to take all the supplements that I do. If you are starting to take a new supplement, check with your healthcare provider. You might be taking medications that are contraindicated. If you are pregnant or about to be, be sure to check with your doctor about the supplements you are taking. Always read the labels and talk to your doctor about dosage.

NICOTINAMIDE RIBOSIDE

Nicotinamide riboside, a precursor to NAD, is a recent addition to the supplements I take. This supplement is quite expensive. You can achieve the same results by drinking hydrogen water. NAD and NADH, what we call a redox couple, are responsible for making energy in the mitochondria. NAD and NADH activate key enzymes such as AMPK that promote energy production and normalize the metabolism to achieve metabolic homeostasis. They regulate functions such as taking up blood sugar, burning fat, and mitochondrial biogenesis.

B COMPLEX

B complex is an important daily supplement that contains the following:

- Thiamin (B_1)
- Riboflavin (B_2)
- Niacin (B_3)
- Pantothenic acid (B_5)
- Pyridoxine (B_6)
- Biotin (B_7)
- Folate, or "folic acid" as a supplement (B_9)
- Cyanocobalamin (B_{12})

Playing a critical role in cellular metabolism, the B vitamins are necessary to metabolize carbohydrates, proteins, and fats. They are an integral part of the energy production pathway and are necessary for optimal cellular function.

CHROMIUM PICOLINATE

I have added chromium picolinate to my daily supplements. Chromium, a trace mineral, plays a role in blood sugar metabolism by enhancing insulin's action. As you know, insulin is responsible for the uptake of blood sugar into the cell. Aging, a poor diet, and a lack of exercise all interfere with the cellular uptake of glucose. Chromium maintains insulin sensitivity by regulating blood sugar levels and normalizing metabolism. When we normalize blood sugar we increase insulin sensitivity, which regulates our appetite and regulates metabolism.

I collaborated on many scientific studies with Dr. Harry Preuss, a tenured professor of physiology, medicine, and pathology at Georgetown Medical Center and author of more than 300 medical papers and more than 200 abstracts. A fellow master of the American College of Nutrition, Dr. Preuss shared my passion for research. One of our joint studies focused on chromium and its ability to normalize blood sugar and increase insulin sensitivity. Too much insulin released into the blood blocks fat burning because fat synthesis and fat burning are highly sensitive to changes in insulin levels that result from eating carbohydrate-rich foods. Small decreases in insulin almost immediately increase fat burning, while increases can activate enzymes that transform glucose into fat.

Other supplements I take each day include:

Alpha-lipoic acid (ALA): Anti-inflammatory, antioxidant; boosts energy by regulating insulin and uptake of glucose by the cells. Increasing the production of the Beauty Molecule, acetylcholine, ALA produces anti-aging effects. ALA is a strong activator of AMPK. ALA is neuroprotective and enhances the health and beauty of the skin.

Known as the universal antioxidant, alpha-lipoic acid is both fat and water soluble, giving it the unique property of being able to reach all parts of the cell. ALA reaches the lipid or fat portions of cells, including the cell plasma membrane and the cytoplasm, the interior of the cell, where water-soluble chemicals reside. This gives lipoic acid a distinct advantage over many antioxidants such as vitamin E, which is only fat soluble, and ascorbic acid, the form of vitamin C that is water soluble.

Part of an enzyme complex known as the pyruvate dehydrogenase complex, ALA is closely involved in the energy production of the cell, enabling the cells to repair themselves in the same way that young cells do. ALA works as a coenzyme in the production of energy by converting carbohydrates into energy (ATP), enhancing our ability to metabolize food into energy. ALA has also been shown to improve cognition and memory.

Its powerful anti-inflammatory properties mean that it can exert many positive effects on a cellular level. It blocks the activation of nuclear factor kappa B (NF-kB) as well as, if not better than, any other antioxidant/anti-inflammatory thus far discovered. Another vital action is lipoic acid's ability to increase the body's sensitivity to insulin, resulting in a decrease in blood sugar levels.

In addition to its function as a powerful antioxidant/anti-inflammatory, alpha-lipoic acid increases the body's ability to take glucose into the cells. ALA works synergistically with CoQ_{10}, carnitine, and acetyl-L-carnitine to protect and rejuvenate the mitochondria. With other antioxidants, ALA raises levels of vitamin C, vitamin E, and glutathione in the cell. ALA is the only antioxidant that can increase glutathione, the most important antioxidant for longevity and overall health. As you have read in chapter 7, glutathione is a cellular tripeptide antioxidant needed for optimal functioning of the immune system. Glutathione is the body's primary water-soluble antioxidant and a major detoxification agent. People with chronic illnesses such as AIDS, cancer, and autoimmune diseases generally have very low levels of glutathione.

Acetyl-L-carnitine: Antioxidant, metabolic enhancer, anti-inflammatory; assists the mitochondria in energy production. This amino acid derivative aids the movement of fatty acids into the mitochondria, where they are converted to energy. Acetyl-L-carnitine improves mitochondrial function in energy production and supports brain health.

Coenzyme Q10: Antioxidant, anti-inflammatory; improves the metabolic profile by increasing AMPK. Another antioxidant in my daily regimen. I take an advanced form known as MitoQ, which is a mitochondria-targeting form of this antioxidant that enhances mitochondrial function and reduces oxidative stress. Q10 has also shown promise in reducing skin wrinkling.

DMAE (Dimethylaminoethanol): A compound that helps synthesize the Beauty Molecule, acetylcholine. Originally a prescription medication, it was used to enhance cognitive function and to treat attention deficit disorder. DMAE is now available in health food stores as a dietary supplement for its potential mood-enhancing and cognitive benefits. Taking DMAE increases muscle tone. When I gave DMAE to my patients, a facial scan showed a more toned appearance, making the patient look younger. Dimethylaminoethanol is a very powerful anti-inflammatory because it stabilizes the cell membrane.

Magnesium: Anti-inflammatory; repairs DNA and RNA, improves muscle function, increases production of AMPK. An essential mineral, magnesium is critical for energy production and is involved in many biochemical reactions in the body, such as making proteins and muscle function. Magnesium is a cofactor for many enzymes, enabling the enzymes to function.

Berberine: Anti-inflammatory; lowers cholesterol and blood pressure. Increases AMPK through the same mechanism as that of metformin. Berberine is extracted from various plants, including goldenseal. It has been studied for years for its potential positive effects on metabolism. Berberine activates cellular switches like AMPK that are so important in maintaining metabolic function. Like chromium, berberine increases the uptake of sugar into the cells, improving sensitivity to insulin and enhancing function of mitochondria. Berberine's effect on metabolism includes enhancing fatty acid oxidation. Berberine is comparable to the prescription drug metformin and is believed to have metformin-like benefits. It is not a prescription drug and is very safe.

Conjugated linoleic acid (CLA): A group of fatty acids found in grass-fed meats and dairy products. CLA has profound effects on metabolism and body composition and will help reestablish the balance of fatty acids. CLA works on a level of gene expression for fatty acid metabolism. I believe CLA prevents unneeded fat storage.

Quercetin: Antioxidant, anti-inflammatory; increases levels of AMPK. Quercetin is one of the flavonoids, present in many fruits, vegetables, and herbs. Quercetin activates cell signaling pathways involved in inflammation and metabolism, making it very important to longevity and health.

Curcumin: The active compound found in the spice turmeric, which has been popular in Indian cuisine for centuries. Turmeric has powerful anti-inflammatory and antioxidant effects and can activate all the various cell signaling mechanisms. Because turmeric is not very well absorbed, I supplement with curcumin, which modulates the molecular targets involved in metabolism and inflammation like AMPK and mTOR.

Urolithin A: A natural metabolite produced by gut bacteria breaking down polyphenols in our food. Though urolithins are not found in food, their precursor polyphenols are. Polyphenols are abundantly found in many fruits and vegetables that contain ellagic acid and/or ellagitannins, including pomegranates, strawberries, blackberries, camu-camu, walnuts, chestnuts, pistachios, pecans, brewed tea, and oak-barrel-aged wines and spirits. Urolithin A has been researched for its effects on normalizing metabolism and improved cellular health. It is anti-inflammatory, activates AMPK, and has positive effects on mitochondrial function. Urolithin A boosts mitochondrial biogenesis. I believe it is critical in maintaining both youth and health.

Vitamin C: In its water-soluble form this antioxidant is known as ascorbic acid. It is critical to the immune system and to the production of collagen and elastin. We have all heard the stories about the scurvy that affected British sailors many years ago. The lack of fresh fruit or vegetables onboard during long ocean voyages resulted in vitamin C deficiency. Scurvy, a serious disease that can be fatal, decimated a great many populations of sailors. It presents as a breakdown of collagen and elastin, with symptoms including bleeding gums. Vitamin C protects us against oxidative stress and is a powerful anti-inflammatory.

I became interested in vitamin C in my early years and had the honor of speaking with Linus Pauling, a Nobel laureate in chemistry, known as one of the twenty greatest scientists of all time. He was an advocate of vitamin C in what he called megadoses. Vitamin C can be taken in fairly high doses because it is not toxic. If we are suffering from colds or viruses, we can take vitamin C as often as every 2 to 3 hours. Vitamin C is extremely important to collagen production. For beautiful skin, adequate vitamin C is a must.

Vitamin C also comes in a fat-soluble form known as ascorbyl palmitate, ideal for using topically on the skin. Your skin will reject water if you pour it on the back of your hand, which is why the water-based form of vitamin C is not recommended as a topical treatment. It is irritating to skin and unstable in topical formulations, discoloring and also losing activity. Reducing inflammation and enhancing elastin and collagen production in the skin, ascorbyl palmitate, thanks to its fat solubility, delivers 5 times the antioxidant power of water-soluble vitamin C.

Vitamins D_3 and K: There is a synergistic interplay between vitamins D and K for bone and cardiovascular health. This combination is part of many biochemical processes in the body, which became obvious during the COVID pandemic. Those with higher levels of vitamin D not only fared better if they had a COVID infection, they also had a lower mortality rate.

Vitamins D and K are fat soluble and play a central role in calcium absorption, vital for bone health. People living in the Northern Hemisphere have lower levels of vitamin D due to decreased exposure to sunlight. As you have read, I recommend sun exposure for a short period each day. Vitamin K plays a role in bone metabolism as well. Both vitamins decrease inflammation and support overall health. Current evidence shows that joint supplementation of vitamins D and K might be more effective than the consumption of either alone for bone or cardiovascular health.

HMB (hydroxymethylbutyrate): Very important in maintaining muscle mass. A hospital study with bedridden patients showed that patients given HMB maintained muscle mass even when immobilized. As we age, the loss of muscle mass and bone density is called frailty, an independent risk factor for death.

EGCG: Polyphenol found in green tea that prevents premature aging and loss of elasticity in skin; increases levels of AMPK through the Beauty Molecule, acetylcholine; and normalizes metabolism. Both antioxidant and anti-inflammatory, EGCG triggers many cell switches that enhance metabolism, making it effective in treating metabolic disorders. EGCG affects AMPK activity and increases insulin sensitivity. I do not take it as an extra supplement, because it is in my tea. If you are not drinking green tea I recommend doing so. It is a powerful supplement that will enhance your youth.

Cinnamon: A delightful spice that enhances any dish. I add ¼ teaspoon to my tea, because it is a proven tool in controlling blood sugar.

MCTs (medium-chain triglycerides): Another daily addition to my tea. MCTs most commonly come from coconut oil. I add 1 tablespoon of C8 MCTs. The C8 means that there are 8 carbons in the chain. Also known as caprylic acid, MCTs are rapidly converted into ketones, an alternative energy source, especially for the brain. Ketones preserve muscle mass as well. Intermittent fasting produces high levels of ketones. The MCTs stabilize our appetite while the ketones have positive effects on the mitochondria and the cell, enhancing mitophagy and autophagy. MCT oil enhances cognitive function, which I appreciate because I do a lot of my writing, reading, and research in the morning hours. This morning ritual of tea, with the polyphenols, cinnamon, and MCT oil to enhance ketone production, all contribute to my energy level and cognitive function.

Omega-3 fish oil: Increases long-chain omega-3s in the brain; reduces inflammatory cytokines, which improves neurotransmitter function.

These fatty acids are vital both to brain function as well as to radiant, youthful, and healthy skin. Incorporating long-chain omega-3s into your diet, whether through high-quality fish oil supplements or by eating cold-water fish such as wild salmon and sardines, you can reduce inflammatory cytokines in the brain, improving the function of neurotransmitters.

The anti-inflammatory power of omega-3 essential fatty acids offers a wide variety of benefits, such as improving attention span, memory, and overall cognitive abilities. The omega-3 fatty acids create and maintain healthful levels of serotonin, a neurotransmitter that affects mood, emotions, appetite, and digestion. The precursor for melatonin, the essential fatty acids help to regulate sleep/wake cycles and the master clock. These fatty acids accelerate the loss of body fat, stabilize blood sugar, lower insulin levels, decrease appetite, and increase energy.

The omega-3s have a role in protecting cardiovascular health, ameliorating chronic skin problems like eczema, increasing immune health, and decreasing the symptoms and severity of rheumatoid arthritis, an autoimmune disease. The omega-3 essential fatty acids reduce inflammation in all organ systems, making them indispensable to physical and mental health. Chronic inflammation can impair the production of anti-inflammatory omega-3 fatty acids, which is another reason to fight inflammation.

As you can see from their many functions, supplements can help your body to operate with efficiency and strength. I know that the supplements I take make a big difference in my energy levels and resilience, and that they support the positive outlook that has empowered me to take on new challenges and persevere.

NEAR-INFRARED LIGHT THERAPY

Another important part of my daily regimen is exposure to red-light infra-red therapy, which is known as photobiomodulation (PBM). This therapy uses red or near-infrared light to stimulate, heal, regenerate, and protect tissue that has been injured, is degenerating, or is at risk of dying. Previously known as low-level laser therapy, it involves the application of red and near-infrared light to injuries or lesions to improve wound and soft tissue healing, reduce inflammation, and give relief for acute and chronic pain.

Photobiomodulation therapy is a safe way to support cellular function. I was happy to discover that skin cells also benefit from light therapy. Using infrared light in pulse mode can penetrate cells deeper below the surface of the skin. In addition to supporting healing during recovery, some studies of this therapy observe an increased production of collagen and elastin in the skin.

The infrared light that is part of the unit I use has a much greater penetration—up to 7 centimeters. The light reaches every organ system because I do the front and back of my body. This therapy affects mitochondrial energy production as well as the function of the mitochondria to activate cellular repair pathways. The red-light and infrared therapy have powerful anti-inflammatory effects and assist by tuning our immune system and turning off pro-inflammatory cytokines.

Infrared-light therapy can suppress nuclear factor kappa B, which signals to produce pro-inflammatory cytokines. Another benefit from infrared and red-light therapy is the improvement of blood flow through the body. Neuroprotective, this therapy protects our brains and slows the process of neurodegeneration. Cognitive decline is a serious problem. If we could delay the onset of Alzheimer's by just months, it would add up to about $300 billion in savings in this country.

BENEFITS OF PHOTOBIOMODULATION
THERAPY

This therapy involves applying red and near-infrared light to the body. It improves wound and soft tissue healing and provides acute and chronic pain relief. In addition, photobiomodulation therapy:

- Enhances production of the neurotransmitter acetylcholine, the Beauty Molecule
- Supports new collagen formation and smooths wrinkles
- Supports joint function and increases mobility
- Accelerates and supports healing during recovery
- Upregulates cell signaling
- Enhances and regulates gene expression

MEDITATION

Meditation is a key part of my morning ritual. Meditation activates the vagus nerve on the parasympathetic side, which oversees an array of crucial bodily functions, including control of mood, immune response, digestion, and heart rate. By activating the parasympathetic system, which governs rest-and-digest functions, meditation produces a calm and relaxed state. Reduction of stress and anxiety are just two of the benefits of stimulating the vagus nerve. Control of mood, immune response, digestion, and heart rate are just a few of the bodily functions the vagus nerve oversees.

The secretion of the Beauty Molecule, acetylcholine, is increased during meditation, which has a powerful effect on cell healing. The increased secretion of acetylcholine during meditation can repair mitochondria. By enhancing the production of acetylcholine and enhancing parasympathetic activation, meditation turns the clock back by increasing energy production and preserving the mitochondria.

I meditate for 20 or 30 minutes every day, which is an excellent way to elevate levels of the Beauty Molecule. Meditating on a daily basis can directly repair the mitochondria and affect physical health. Meditation increases vagal tone, resulting in secretion of the Beauty Molecule, which creates an anti-inflammatory environment.

START THE DAY WITH GREEN TEA

The next part of my morning regimen is to enjoy a delicious cup of tea. Tea is a rich source of the polyphenols that help to normalize the metabolism and upregulate the master metabolic molecule, AMPK. I particularly like white tea with jasmine, because the jasmine flowers impart a lovely fragrance and relaxing element to the tea. Instead of cream, milk, or sweetener, I add C8 medium-chain triglycerides (MCTs). Although there are four different types of MCTs, C8 MCT oil provides the most health benefits. Supplementing with C8 MCT oil can potentially improve mental clarity, energy levels, and influence fat loss.

As fans of the keto diet know, the C8 MCTs produce ketones very rapidly. Via my tea, it upregulates the master metabolic activator AMPK. By pushing my body into ketosis, it provides an alternative fuel for the body, especially the brain. Ketones, molecules that provide energy and act as fuel, are also an anti-inflammatory.

In addition to the medium-chain triglyceride, I also take a teaspoon of extra-virgin olive oil, which is known to upregulate the sirtuin genes, known as the longevity genes, far better than many of the expensive products, like resveratrol, currently on the market, which have questionable effectiveness.

I add ¼ teaspoon of cinnamon to the tea because it stabilizes blood sugar for several hours.

Green tea is rich in phytochemicals, which become very active within our bodies. The antioxidant properties of green tea derive from a group of polyphenols called catechins, which neutralize free radicals and reduce oxidative stress. Green tea has been associated with reduced heart disease, and may improve blood vessel function and reduce blood pressure. Green tea has been found to enhance metabolism and promote metabolism of fats, making it easier for individuals to lose excess body fat. Green tea can inhibit the growth of negative bacteria in the mouth and improve oral health.

Green tea's compounds are known to be very active in the central nervous system. Although it contains caffeine, it will not cause the jitters often associated with caffeine thanks to the presence of the amino acid L-theanine. This amino acid improves cognitive function and exerts a calming effect, bestowing alertness without the negative effects of stimulants.

There is excellent data showing that the polyphenols in green tea, particularly EGCG (epigallocatechin gallate), have anticancer properties, reduce inflammation, and improve insulin sensitivity, which is helpful in preventing type 2 diabetes

In my first book, published 20 years ago, I talked about the necessity of carefully controlling blood sugar and insulin, which has always been the hallmark of my dietary advice. Now many people are writing about this, as if it were a recent discovery. The world has finally realized that elevated blood sugar and insulin levels are a fast track to accelerated aging and a host of chronic and often deadly diseases.

TIME-RESTRICTED EATING AND MY PERSONAL ROUTINE AT MEALS

I have been following the time-restricted eating program intermittently for more than 2 years. I do not follow my tea with breakfast. I fast all day until I have my first meal sometime between 5 and 6 p.m. Later in the evening I have a snack to ensure I have adequate daily protein, which is especially important if I have been very physically active.

One of the major benefits of time-restricted eating is the maintenance of very low blood sugar and insulin, which has a powerful anti-inflammatory effect. Going into ketosis adds anti-inflammatory benefits and positive results on metabolism.

Of course, protein plays an important role in my daily meal choices. As I have said, we age on the days that we do not get enough protein. That is why I start my first meal of the day with wild salmon, which is one of the best forms of protein available. Other good sources of protein include free-range poultry, eggs, and grass-fed meats. Animal and plant proteins are composed of about twenty common amino acids. Proteins that do not have all the amino acids are known as incomplete proteins. Having all of the requisite amino acids, salmon is a complete protein.

Another hugely important benefit of eating salmon is increased levels of nitric oxide. Rich in the carotenoid astaxanthin, salmon is king when it comes to radiant skin. Astaxanthin also reduces the risk of developing macular degeneration.

Salmon is a great source of long-chain omega-3 essential fatty acids, which are well known for their ability to protect us from and inhibit inflammation. We now know the importance of the essential fatty acids and their ability to protect the cells of our heart. Omega-3s act as natural antidepressants and keep the skin radiant.

TAURINE

Wild salmon and many other kinds of fish and meat contain high levels of an amino acid, the building block of protein, called taurine. Taurine has many functions in the body, including working as a neurotransmitter in the brain.

A study published in the journal *Science*, led by Columbia researchers and involving dozens of researchers in the field of aging around the world, had some remarkable results. The study found that taurine supplements can slow down the aging process in worms, mice, and monkeys and can even extend the healthy lifespans of middle-aged mice by up to 12 percent, according to the leader of the study, Vijay Yadav, Ph.D., assistant professor of genetics and development at Columbia University's Vagelos College of Physicians and Surgeons. For the past 25 years, scientists have been trying to find factors that not only let us live longer, but also increase health span, the time we remain healthy in our old age. This study suggests that taurine could be an elixir of life within us that helps us live longer and healthier lives.

Taurine, an antioxidant and anti-inflammatory, can lower blood pressure and is protective against cardiovascular disease, especially congestive heart failure. Taurine plays an important role in building bone, which prevents osteoporosis and subsequent bone frailty. In addition, taurine levels have been found to correlate with immune and nervous system functions. In short, taurine regulates all these processes that decline with age. Following the anti-inflammatory diet and eating salmon regularly is a great way to naturally increase taurine levels.

In addition to aiding in the digestion of fats, taurine is involved in the maintenance of ions that help to keep energy concentrations in the cell working correctly. Taurine demonstrates multiple cellular functions, including a central role as a neurotransmitter. Taurine deficiency is associated with depression, as well as with anxiety and other behavioral problems seen in children. Taurine has been used in the treatment of severe fatigue and alcoholism. This amino acid has been shown to inhibit cancerous tumors and prevents against oxidative stress.

SALADS, VEGETABLES, AND FRUIT

Green salads are another major component of my daily diet. A great source of phytochemicals, salads are an excellent vehicle for extra-virgin olive oil. The combination of salad with extra-virgin olive oil is a source of nitrates, which promote the synthesis of nitric oxide. Seeds and nuts are delicious additions to any salad. Fresh lemon juice is an excellent addition to extra-virgin olive oil in dressings.

Salads are healthful for many reasons. When a salad enters the digestive tract, the bacteria in the gut and mouth can convert nitrates to nitrite. That means that the worst thing we can do is to use mouthwash, because doing so destroys this conversion, negatively affecting our nitric oxide levels, which leads to increasing the risk of certain diseases— high blood pressure, for example. The benefits of increasing nitric oxide production in our bodies with dietary sources like salmon can have positive effects on the brain, the cardiovascular system, and the immune system.

I enjoy servings of all of the cruciferous vegetables, such as broccoli, watercress, broccoli rabe, cauliflower, and many more. Using fresh lemon juice as a finish makes these vegetables brighter and more delicious.

Blueberries, another mainstay of my meal, confer a number of health benefits. Blueberries contain an antioxidant called anthocyanin, responsible for the deep blue color. Anthocyanins help to neutralize free radicals and reduce oxidative stress. Blueberries are important for improved heart health, and may help lower blood pressure and reduce the risk of heart disease. The anthocyanins are protective of brain cells. Another example of the brain-beauty connection, anthocyanins are also protective of the skin.

Thanks to their anti-inflammatory power, blueberries reduce the overall inflammation burden in the body, reducing our risk for a number of diseases. Like the antioxidants in green tea, blueberries increase insulin sensitivity, reducing blood sugar levels, which is important in the prevention of diabetes and a host of degenerative diseases and conditions. Blueberries also contain a large amount of fiber, which feeds the gut bacteria and aids digestion.

Other antioxidants present in blueberries include lutein and zeaxanthin, which are beneficial for eye health, helping to prevent macular degeneration. Studies have shown that the antioxidants from the phytochemicals in blueberries reduce the risk of cancer. Nothing is more delicious than a bowl of fresh blueberries. Their myriad health and beauty benefits make them a vital part of my daily meal and the anti-inflammatory diet.

The remaining chapters in *The Beauty Molecule* explore strategies for fighting inflammation; increasing longevity; and enhancing, saving, or restoring the youthful radiance of your skin. Of course, you are already trying to adopt the anti-inflammatory diet, which is such an important step. I decided to highlight the way to eat in part 1 of this book. In the following chapters, you will learn about light and your biological clock, movement and exercise, meditation, intermittent fasting, topicals, and more on supplements.

Adding so many life-changing practices to your already hectic life may seem a high mountain to climb. You might risk overwhelming yourself if you try to do too much to start. You do not want to begin strong and find yourself dropping strategies because of lack of time and will. I suggest you ease into living an inflammation-fighting lifestyle. The changes you experience will feel so great you will be encouraged to try more.

One strategy might have special appeal for you because it addresses a particular problem or need. You may realize that you are addicted to junk food, and that cleaning up your diet might be your greatest challenge. Intermittent fasting could be a way to get back on track and to boost your energy. If falling asleep is challenging for you, you will want to adjust your biological clock. Maybe you are sedentary and need to get moving, even if it means making sure to get up and stand every hour. When you have noticed you are losing muscle mass and are not happy about the changes you see in your face and body, the twice-a-week, 20-minute resistance workout could help you shape up and give you more energy. If you are stressed-out, anxious, and depressed, meditation could calm you down and lift your spirits. The chapters on topicals and supplements, areas of special interest to me, will introduce you to the active ingredients to look for in skin-care products and supplements you can take that will support the Beauty Molecule and combat inflammation.

I advise you to commit to start by trying one of the strategies. When you incorporate one or two strategies into your life, you will notice a positive difference and will want to try more. If a strategy does not deliver what you expect, see if another works better for you. As soon as a practice becomes a habit, move on to another strategy. Or you might be ready to jump right in and try adding all the strategies to your day.

Regardless of how you approach the strategies, you are making a conscious decision to do what has proven to be effective in increasing your lifespan and health span as well as creating smooth, supple, and glowing skin.

10

SEEING THE LIGHT

WHEN I FIRST LEARNED ABOUT the miraculous benefits of phototherapy, also known as light therapy, I knew that we had a therapeutic intervention with incomparable protective functions. My first exposure was during my internship in pediatrics at Yale University's New Haven Hospital. I was beginning my internship, which traditionally starts at the end of June. I was told that I would be on call on June 23, which happened to be my birthday. Assigned to a very busy service at the hospital, the intensive care unit for newborns, I prepared myself for the long 36 hours ahead.

Pediatric residents were traditionally assigned to the delivery room, which was housed in the Grace-New Haven Hospital, the older section of the hospital. That morning being no exception, I was called in to assist in a difficult delivery. If the newborn is in trouble during a difficult delivery, we often need to initiate life support measures. The baby was experiencing respiratory difficulties in this case. Accompanied by my senior resident, we administered oxygen. I happened to glance at my watch and noticed that not only was it my birthday, but also that the time was 11:31 a.m., the exact hour and minute of my own birth, which had also taken place in that very delivery room many years earlier.

After returning to the newborn special care unit, I noticed a group of babies receiving a light from a device suspended above them. Intrigued by what the light could be, I asked the senior resident about it. He explained that when babies are born prematurely, or sometimes even for those with full-term, normal deliveries, they can have difficulty breaking down a substance in their blood known as bilirubin, a yellowish pigment produced during the decomposition of red blood cells. Bilirubin gives the skin and the whites of the eyes a visible yellow cast, known as infant jaundice, which is more than just a cosmetic problem. These elevated levels, known as bilirubin anemia, can cause brain damage. Normally, the body is able to remove the bilirubin by breaking it up into nontoxic precursors, which pass through the liver and are excreted from the body. When the liver of newborns cannot detoxify the bilirubin, bilirubin anemia results. The traditional treatment at the time had been to perform an exchange transfusion of blood. This involved repeatedly withdrawing small amounts of blood and replacing it with donor blood, which would dilute the bilirubin and, unfortunately, the maternal antibodies. The exchange transfusion was a 4-hour procedure.

Sister Jean Ward, a nurse at Rochford Hospital in Essex, United Kingdom, in 1956, routinely took newborns out into the sunlight. This instinctive action ultimately led to the breakthrough of the inadvertent discovery of phototherapy as a successful treatment. Physicians noticed that babies exposed to sunlight had reduced jaundice. When babies were taken out into the sunlight, the bilirubin anemia resolved much more quickly than in those babies who were not exposed to light. Blood studies showed that the level of bilirubin decreased with exposure to sunlight.

This discovery inspired Dr. R. J. Cremer to create the first phototherapy machine, designed to treat premature infants for jaundice. His device consisted of fluorescent bulbs that were placed over the infant's crib. Dr. Cremer's study of 11 infants who had been treated with phototherapy found that 9 of the babies experienced reduced levels of bilirubin, which eliminated the need for the exchange transfusions.

In the United States, Dr. Jerold Lucey of the University of Vermont conducted a landmark randomized clinical trial, published in *Pediatrics* in 1968. The protocol for the jaundiced children did not change. Even after the publication of Dr. Lucey's study on phototherapy, the procedure was not accepted by physicians until about a decade later, during which time exchange transfusions continued to be the primary treatment.

Today phototherapy has been refined using LEDs (light-emitting diodes), sometimes in a blanket to treat these newborn children. Witnessing the use of phototherapy at the Yale New Haven Hospital left a deep impression upon me. Learning about the power of light therapy and seeing firsthand how it could be an effective, noninvasive treatment of a very severe problem was inspiring.

I was extremely interested in exploring if the concept of mitochondrial repair was the basis for the therapeutic effects of light on neurodegeneration. My next exposure to phototherapy came from a published article by an English physician, Dr. Gordon Dougal in the United Kingdom, which caught my attention.

Dr. Dougal was working with near-infrared therapy. Near-infrared light is not visible to the eye, falling from the invisible part of the electromagnetic light spectrum between 700 and 1,200 nanometers. Dr. Dougal was doing animal studies on cognitive decline. He was irradiating mice suffering from Alzheimer's disease with near-infrared light at a frequency of 1,072 nanometers. Although infrared light is invisible to the eye, this in no way diminishes its efficacy. Near-infrared light with its long wavelengths can penetrate deeply into soft tissues, muscles, joints, and bones. Visible red light reaches a depth of only about a quarter of an inch. Red light is on the visible part of the light spectrum, between 530 and 700 nanometers on the electromagnetic scale. The longer the wavelength, the deeper the penetration to deliver energy to cells. That is why red light is used to treat the surface of the skin.

After studying the literature as well as witnessing the actual effects of infrared, Dr. Dougal believed there could possibly be benefits in irradiating these mice with infrared, especially at 1,072 nanometers, because this frequency can uniquely transmit through water. Since the cell is composed, in large part, of water, this frequency would give greater penetration.

After a few weeks of treatment, Dr. Dougal observed that the Alzheimer's-inflicted mice were actually gaining back cognitive function. They were able to function as normal mice when it came to food intake and movement. After a short time, Dr. Dougal looked at human studies using near-infrared light.

He designed a helmet known as PBM-T that contained multiple LEDs specific for the frequency of 1,072 nanometers. The helmet had to be carefully planned and constructed because LEDs create heat. Heat can cause changes in the light frequency, which had to be very specific. He incorporated fourteen small fans in the helmet to keep the temperature down and to maintain the desired 1,072-nanometer frequency, delivering infrared light deep into the brain for 6-minute treatment cycles of 1,368 joules of energy.

Scientists discovered that photoreceptors absorb light in the cell—specifically in the mitochondria. The infrared light stimulates the mitochondria, which, as you know, generate most of the chemical energy needed to power the biochemical reactions of the cells. This, in turn, leads to a rise in the level of the organic compound ATP, necessary to provide the energy to drive processes in living cells and help nerve cells to repair. Unfortunately, ATP is markedly decreased in dementia patients.

In addition, near-infrared light treatment can increase levels of nitric oxide, affecting blood flow in the brain by improving the flexibility of the membrane that lines the inside of blood vessels. This widens blood vessels, which enables more oxygen to reach the white matter deep in the brain.

PUTTING IT TO THE TEST

A family in the United States approached Dr. Dougal and asked him to see their father who, although only 57 years of age, was suffering from Alzheimer's. He had lost his independence and his ability to speak, a condition known as aphasia. Dr. Dougal arranged for the patient to wear the PBM-T helmet for 6 minutes each day.

Within 2 weeks of beginning therapy, the patient showed great improvement and started to speak once again. After another few weeks, the patient's independence was somewhat restored. He was able to drive his car again and run small errands.

Inspired by the success of the treatments, Dr. Dougal continued his studies using near-infrared light for treating neurological issues. Many neurological problems such as traumatic brain injury can improve with exposure to near-infrared light therapy. One of the most impressive findings I have seen is the improvements in patients with Parkinson's disease. When treated with various frequencies of near-infrared light on a daily basis, the patients experienced a marked diminishment in the symptoms of this debilitating disease.

Because of the brain-beauty connection, the strong correlation between the skin and the brain, I was eager to speak to Dr. Dougal about his ongoing research. I knew that certain pharmaceuticals used to treat mental disorders and conditions had a visible and often positive effect on the skin. This near-infrared light at 1,072 nanometers was having such a powerful healing effect for people with brain injuries, cognitive decline, or progressive degenerative diseases of the brain like Alzheimer's. I wondered, What benefits would it provide to the skin?

Dr. Dougal was kind enough to speak with me about his research, as well as provide me with some devices that contained LEDs. Eager to get started, I began applying the near-infrared therapy to skin. Within a matter of days, the subject reported a pulling sensation in the skin. We could observe that the migration of the fibroblasts to repair the skin was taking place. The skin appeared more radiant and was firmer. Later studies showed that elastin and collagen were regenerating.

A tremendous amount of research has been done since 2000. We now know, beyond a doubt, that light therapy has tremendous therapeutic benefits in both disease models and in improving overall health.

THE SUN ALSO RISES

In addition to the extensive benefits of near-infrared therapy, my studies focused on the sun as a source of powerful natural healing properties. The sun has the ability to increase levels of melatonin, which is a powerful antioxidant in the mitochondria as well as a hormone the brain produces in response to darkness. Melatonin helps to regulate the timing of your 24-hour internal clock, known as circadian rhythms. Circadian rhythms are physical, mental, and behavioral changes that follow a 24-hour cycle. These natural processes respond primarily to light and dark and affect most living things, including animals, plants, and microbes. Acetylcholine, the Beauty Molecule, is closely involved with our circadian rhythm.

ABUNDANT BENEFITS OF NEAR-INFRARED THERAPY

Near-infrared light falls on the spectrum of light barely visible to the eye, with wavelengths falling between 700 and 2,500 nanometers. The therapy has been shown to:

- Provide anti-aging benefits
- Boost metabolism
- Recharge mitochondria
- Reduce inflammation
- Rejuvenate the skin
- Increase energy
- Reduce body fat
- Improve flexibility
- Lessen joint and muscle pain
- Provide pain relief
- Improve circulation
- Accelerate wound healing
- Reduce recovery time after a workout

These far-reaching benefits include many of the goals of my program, and more.

The daily changes in the release of acetylcholine are controlled by the release of the cholinergic enzymes and the number of acetylcholine-activated receptors in various organ systems. The highest levels of acetylcholine occur during the most active portion of the day, when the enzyme that creates acetylcholine (acetyltransferase) is upregulated. As the evening approaches, acetylcholinesterase decreases the availability of acetylcholine. The receptors for acetylcholine are at their most sensitive and highest levels when acetylcholine is at its lowest secretion.

THE MASTER CLOCK

A master clock in the brain coordinates all the biological clocks in a living thing, keeping the clocks in sync. In vertebrate animals, including humans, the master clock is a group of about 20,000 neurons that form a structure called the suprachiasmatic nucleus, or SCN. The SCN, located in the brain's hypothalamus, receives direct input from the eyes. In the master clock, the Beauty Molecule interacts in the central nervous system and influences the circadian rhythm.

Important genes, such as the period and cryptochrome, are involved with the master clock. These genes code for proteins that increase in the cell's nucleus at night and decrease during the day, which may activate feelings of wakefulness, alertness, and tiredness.

Signals from the environment also affect circadian rhythms. For instance, exposure to light at a different time of day can reset when the body turns on period and cryptochrome genes.

Our circadian rhythms are triggered either by light exposure or the lack of it. When the body is activated by exposure to light, the acetylcholine release readies the body for activity by controlling many organ systems and hormones. The Beauty Molecule regulates all organ systems by means of the master clock, determining energy level, brain activity, skin radiance, and muscle tone. When you awaken in the morning, your exposure to the light is critical in activating the master clock.

Melatonin is closely tied to our master clock's governing of the circadian rhythm. It must be produced at the right times. Acetylcholine controls production of melatonin. When the amount of light reaching our retina decreases, the body begins making melatonin, which is secreted by the pineal gland in the brain into our circulation as we sleep. It is taken up by the cells and then later by the mitochondria, where free radicals are being produced.

The most important function of melatonin may well be its ability to scavenge harmful free radicals. Melatonin provides on-site protection against oxidative damage to cells. Melatonin acts as a primary nonenzymatic, anti-oxidative defense against the devastating actions of the extremely reactive hydroxyl radical, the most damaging of all free radicals. When melatonin quenches the free radicals, the integrity of the mitochondria is maintained.

If we do not live in synchronicity with the master clock and instead keep late night hours with high levels of light exposure, our melatonin production is suppressed. You need to be aware of how important it is to maximize production of this powerful antioxidant. When we sleep, a meager 5 percent of melatonin is produced by the pineal gland. We need darkness to foster its production. Any form of light during this period shuts down the pineal gland's production of melatonin. The melatonin produced in the brain is circulated through the body, and a certain amount reaches the mitochondria.

Light exposure during daytime hours is needed for this production. Our best source is from exposure to the sun. Sunlight includes different parts of the electromagnetic spectrum. In addition to visible light, a part of the electromagnetic spectrum coming from the sun is not visible. This is infrared light. To maximize exposure to the visible and infrared spectrum, we need to get into the sun immediately upon awakening as well as at sunset. The light interacts with our retinas and sends signals to adjust our master clock for optimal melatonin production. Exposing ourselves to the sunlight at these times, we gain the greatest benefits when the sun is not strong enough to do damage. The aim is to avoid the harmful ultraviolet rays that damage our skin, causing wrinkles, loss of firmness, and the dangers of skin cancer.

As you learned in the discussion about Dr. Dougal's groundbreaking research, the infrared portion of the invisible spectrum, especially the near infrared, can penetrate the body to a depth of up to 3 inches. Although this light is not part of the visible light spectrum, we can feel it as warmth on the skin. This feeling of warmth confirms that we are receiving infrared wavelengths. This highly penetrating form of electromagnetic radiation can directly stimulate the production of melatonin in the mitochondria, enabling its superior antioxidant properties to protect this highly important part of the cell. Near-infrared light also reflects off trees and grass. While sitting under a tree, you can get near-infrared light that will enhance your levels of melatonin and protect the mitochondria. Just remember not to wear your sunglasses during this time. Your retina needs to absorb the light.

EARLY TO BED, EARLY TO RISE

It is important to our health and beauty to have strategies that will align our schedule with our master clock when possible.

There are two main strategies to influence the production of melatonin:

- Darkness at night when you sleep
- Exposure to near-infrared light during daylight hours

You should not need to take melatonin supplements at bedtime, because the pineal gland will secrete melatonin to help you to fall asleep. You need darkness when you sleep to foster the production of melatonin. Any form of light during sleep shuts down the pineal gland's production of melatonin.

Limiting your exposure to bright light after sunset is the ultimate goal. If you have to work with devices like your laptop or phone, or like falling asleep with the television on, set the screens on low intensity. Wearing blue blocker glasses can help to reduce exposure to light.

INFRARED THERAPY AT HOME

Hundreds of different light boxes and panels are available online for red and near-infrared therapy. More red-light panels seem to be out there than near-infrared-light equipment. Some panels mix red and near-infrared light. There are even handheld devices. Do research before you invest in equipment, and be sure to follow directions. Overexposure is not a good thing.

Infrared saunas are also available. Some are large wooden structures, but there are small individual saunas available as well. You can have one of your own at home to use on a regular basis. Many spas, wellness centers, gyms, and chiropractors' offices offer infrared saunas to their clients.

11

DEEP BREATHING AND MEDITATION

MEDITATION, YOGA, SINGING, CHANTING, BREATH work, and massage are all tried-and-true methods of stimulating the vagus nerve, a simple and enjoyable process. When you stimulate the vagus nerve, you reduce stress and anxiety. If you feel tense or restless, you can manage the jitters simply by taking a few deep breaths.

Stimulating the vagus nerve is important in the fight against inflammation. The vagus nerve, an information superhighway, is our direct communication with the nervous system. The main component of the parasympathetic nervous system, the vagus nerve establishes a connection between the brain and the gastrointestinal tract and sends information about the state of the inner organs to the brain through afferent (incoming) nerve fibers. As you have learned, the vagus nerve oversees many crucial bodily functions, including control of mood, immune response, digestion, and heart rate. And the Beauty Molecule, acetylcholine, is the neurotransmitter that activates the parasympathetic nervous system.

THE IMPORTANCE OF BREATH

There is a reason you take a deep breath before you are about to do something challenging. When you inhale deeply, the oxygen supply to your brain increases and endorphins are released that make you more alert. If you hold your breath, you can activate the fight-or-flight response. A deep breath stretches the fibers around your lungs. That sensory input travels up your vagus nerve to your brain and triggers a deep exhalation, which activates the parasympathetic nervous system to calm you down. Diaphragmatic breathing creates a feedback loop that stimulates a relaxation response.

Deep breathing helps to improve the balance in your autonomic nervous system by releasing the Beauty Molecule, acetylcholine, the chief neurotransmitter of the parasympathetic branch of the autonomic nervous system, to stimulate the vagus nerve. Building a deep-breathing regimen into your day will improve your heart rate variability, and that will increase your longevity.

An excellent and illuminating study, "Breath of Life: The Respiratory Vagal Stimulation Model of Contemplative Activity," published in *Frontiers in Human Neuroscience* (https://www.ncbi.nlm.nih.gov/pmc/articles/PMC6189422/), reports that contemplative practices, such as meditation and yoga, confer beneficial effects including increased physical health, mental health, and cognitive performance. The study demonstrated that what these various contemplative activities have in common is attentively guided or regulated breathing. This respiratory discipline may explain the physical and mental benefits of contemplative activities through changes in autonomic balance.

What resonated with me from this study is the neurophysiological model the authors propose to describe how these specific respiration styles operate by stimulating the vagus nerve. The vagus nerve is the prime candidate for explaining the effects of contemplative practices on health, mental health, and cognition. That is not all. As you know, studies have shown that stimulating the vagus nerve also influences physical health by suppressing inflammation.

When we upregulate the vagus nerve, increasing vagal tone, the Beauty

Molecule, acetylcholine, is secreted on a cellular level and repairs mitochondria. The mitochondria control much more than just energy production—as crucial as that is. The mitochondria are responsible for homeostasis on a systemic level.

With meditation, you promote the production of the Beauty Molecule, acetylcholine, which begins to repair your mitochondria. When you meditate daily, the acetylcholine secreted restructures the mitochondria into a healthy oval shape.

DEEP, CALMING BREATH

Normally you take 10 to 14 breaths a minute. When you practice deep breathing, you aim for 5 to 7 breaths a minute. There is nothing complicated about diaphragmatic breathing. You can practice deep breathing anytime, anyplace. Unless you exaggerate your in-out breath, no one has to know what you are doing. You can practice deep breathing while standing on line, sitting in a waiting room chair, or preparing dinner.

A step-by-step guide:

- Take a slow, deep breath through your nose until you cannot inhale anymore. You usually breathe from the top of your lungs. Visualize filling up your lungs from bottom to top. The lower part of your lungs, above the navel, should fill up like a balloon.
- Slowly release air through pursed lips, constricting your abs as you do so.
- Counting can focus your attention. Try inhaling to a count of 5 and exhaling to a count of 5.
- As you become accustomed to deep breathing, aim to take twice as long to exhale as you did to inhale.

Practicing deep breathing every day will help to restore balance in your body. If you find yourself feeling stressed or panicky, simply do three in-and-out deep-breathing cycles. That alone will calm you.

What was once anecdotal evidence of increased energy from those who meditated can now be ascribed to mitochondrial repair. Those who meditate consistently will tell you that after a few months they not only feel better, but they also look younger. They have normalized their metabolism and repaired their mitochondria.

FROM DEEP BREATHING TO MEDITATION

Controlled breathing is often a component of meditation, a contemplative exercise aimed at changing your mental state. Meditation involves both the mind and body. Practicing meditation has been shown to produce changes in cognition, sensory perception, emotion, brain chemicals and circuitry, and autonomic nervous system activity.

Meditation grants us the power to access our autonomic nervous system to turn off the switch for cellular inflammation, by acting as an internal transmitter. When we meditate, we activate the parasympathetic side of the autonomic nervous system. The vagus nerve sends a signal resulting in the secretion of acetylcholine along our parasympathetic nervous system. In turn, this activates our rest-and-digest hormones. When acetylcholine is released during meditation it has many functions, chief of which is the activation of AMPK, enabling us to maintain metabolic health and slow the aging process. As AMPK is activated, there is also a decrease in inflammation, chronic inflammation in particular. Meditation also works in tandem with deep breathing.

The practice of meditation is one of the most important strategies we have for activating the release of the Beauty Molecule. As you know, the increase in the secretion of acetylcholine results in reduction of inflammation, which is our goal. Because of this effect, meditation is a superb strategy for implementing our quest for health, beauty, and a long and happy life.

The West has been late to recognize the benefits of meditation, which are as numerous as they are diverse. Though meditation has been a tradition in East and South Asia for centuries, we in the West have taken an interest in the contemplative tradition in the past 50 years. During the 1970s, Dr. Herbert Benson at Harvard began studying the effects of meditation on the mind and body. He published his findings in a popular book,

The Relaxation Response, in which he presented scientific evidence of the benefits of meditation, including an increase in the density of brain cells in the hippocampus, critical to the formation of memory.

Much research has been done since. Today many scientific studies document the physical, mental, and spiritual benefits of meditation. First and foremost, these studies confirm what happens in your body when you meditate and that these benefits occur on a cellular level.

Meditation has been shown to lower heart rate, blood pressure, and cholesterol. Meditation's significant anti-inflammatory effect is of particular interest to me because the Beauty Molecule is released during meditation. Decreases in inflammatory markers such as cortisol, C-reactive protein, and pro-inflammatory cytokines have been consistently reported.

MEDITATION AND THE STRESS HORMONES

Studies have shown that practicing meditation decreases stress and lowers the levels of cortisol, epinephrine (adrenaline), and norepinephrine (noradrenalin), which are all stress hormones.

Elevated cortisol levels produce significant negative effects that include:

- Increased inflammation
- Increased insulin secretion
- Increased appetite
- Storage of fat, particularly in the abdomen
- Death of brain cells. High levels of stress shrink the brain and other organs.
- Destruction of the immune system
- Decreased muscle mass
- Accelerated aging
- Increased risk of acne flare-ups. Acne is a systemic inflammatory disease, and stress precipitates acne breakouts.
- Progressive loss of protein

Cortisol is a death hormone that increases as we age. Any good strategy that lowers your cortisol levels will make a big contribution to your health and well-being. As I often point out, our skin is an unfortunate victim of elevated cortisol levels, becoming thin and fragile, losing its tensile strength and elasticity.

Elevated cortisol levels can lead to protein loss, and collagen is the most abundant protein in the body. The loss of protein results in the progressive thinning and reduction of collagen in the body, including the skin, primarily caused by inhibited collagen synthesis. Too much cortisol is catabolic; that is, it breaks down tissue. For example, an excess of cortisol, an adrenal hormone, removes the protein from the skin and shuttles it into muscle tissue to prepare the body for the fight-or-flight adrenal response. This thinner skin takes on a more translucent appearance, resulting in prominent blood vessels and visible veins.

Meditation has been shown to create a sense of peace and balance that contributes to emotional well-being and health. Regular practitioners of meditation report that they feel calmer, that they think with more clarity, and that they have more physical and mental energy after each session of meditation. The emotional benefits of meditation have a direct impact on maintaining balance in your body. The positive emotional and mental effects of meditation include:

- Gaining perspective on stressful situations
- Building skills to manage stress
- Focusing on the present
- Reducing negative emotions
- Increasing patience and tolerance

A study published on PubMed points to the accumulation of evidence-based research that proves the direct and indirect benefits of meditation. It has been found that the practice of meditation triggers neurotransmitters that modulate psychological disorders such as anxiety.

Science is proving that meditation is an ideal antidote highly recommended for stress management. Anxiety is rampant in our culture. Anxiety disorders affect approximately 40 million adults in the United States in a given year. Meditation could help to lower these alarming statistics.

MEDITATION AND YOUR SKIN

An emerging field of research called psychodermatology studies the interaction between mind and skin by looking at the effects of emotions on the skin as well as disorders that have skin manifestations. I witness this mind/body connection often. My patients who suffer from eczema (atopic dermatitis) under stressful situations will often break out in redness during my physical examination. Meditation addresses the underlying issues that exacerbate these skin problems.

Your skin is the target of an acute and chronic stress response, which can be mitigated by the increased production of the anti-inflammatory Beauty Molecule, acetylcholine, in your skin. Your skin is the first to show physical signs of stress. By bridging the gap between your emotional and mental states with your overall health, meditation reduces negative emotions. Meditation reduces stress fear, worry, and anxiety, which are often the root causes of skin problems.

Deep breathing while meditating adds oxygen to the skin, which boosts cellular health. The increased release of acetylcholine during meditation results in healthful relaxation and widening of the vessels by stimulating the production of nitric oxide, which is responsible for the health of your circulatory system and enhances brain function. The effect of nitric oxide explains the radiance that results from meditation and the 3-day anti-inflammatory diet. The increased oxygen rejuvenates your skin, improving your complexion, reducing wrinkles, and slowing down the aging process from the inside out. In addition, meditation helps to reduce muscular tension in the face, relaxing the muscles that can cause wrinkles. To look your best before any event, meditate to create a beautiful glow. If you want to have fresh, youthful skin, add meditation to your daily routine.

FATHER JAMES TURNS BACK THE CLOCK

When it comes to one of the most fascinating examples of the far-reaching and miraculous effects of meditation, a patient of mine deserves top billing. You met Father James in chapter 3. He had agreed to meet with me for a follow-up visit when he returned to the US.

I was delighted to see that his health and overall appearance were significantly improved. He looked better nourished. Having seen his cardiologist, he was happy to report that the pericarditis, the SARS-related inflammation around his heart, was stable. He had followed my advice. Upon his return to the UK, he took a position as a vicar with a small parish church 30 minutes west of London rather than continuing his far-flung missionary work.

He explained that in addition to his daily prayers, he had adopted the ancient tradition of meditation, also every day. He felt it was helping him both physically and spiritually.

Although he was no longer working in the harsh conditions of developing countries, his workload had not diminished. After his return to the UK, he began working as a chaplain for two large hospitals under the auspices of the National Health Service. Though he loved the work and relished each day, he was exhausted by the time he returned to the States a few years later, after COVID restrictions were lifted. Father James had been working 12-hour shifts in the hospitals almost 7 days a week, giving help to the patients and families during the pandemic. I was amazed that he had not contracted the illness himself from his prolonged and constant exposure.

As we sat and talked, I marveled at his drastically improved appearance. Father James not only looked 10 years younger, his calm and confident demeanor radiated a strong sense of well-being despite the fact that he had been working long hours in a hospital setting. I can attest that such a setting is not conducive to relaxation. Working at a hospital is highly stressful and anxiety-inducing, especially during a health crisis. Father James's constitution and sense of well-being had not diminished despite the long hours, disquieting and taxing environment, emotional toll of dealing with hourly trauma and stress, his age, and his heart disease. In fact, he was more robust and upbeat than he had been the last time I saw him. His transformation provided me with my first glimpse of the power of meditation.

Although I was amazed by such a dramatic turnaround in a patient, I realized that meditation was a known factor in increasing vagal tone. Meditation can stimulate the vagus nerve, increasing vagal tone and positive emotions.

MEDITATION AND THE BRAIN

When we meditate, there are direct and powerful effects in the brain. These include an increase in brain-derived neurotrophic factor, or BDNF. Brain-derived neurotrophic factor is a protein found in the central nervous system involved in neurological changes related to learning and memory. BDNF helps the brain develop new connections, repair failing brain cells, and protect healthy brain cells. As we age, our BDNF decreases, negatively affecting our cognitive abilities. Healthful levels of BDNF are vital in preventing cognitive decline and diseases such as multiple sclerosis and Alzheimer's, Parkinson's, and Huntington's disease.

BDNF creates neurogenesis, especially in the hippocampus, where memory is stored. The title of a study published in the *Annals of the New York Academy of Sciences* is the question, "Does Meditation Enhance Cognition and Brain Plasticity?" The authors recognize that meditation has various health benefits, including the possibility of preserving cognition and preventing dementia. The authors go on to acknowledge that studies have shown that meditation may affect multiple pathways that could play a role in brain aging and mental fitness. The study reports that meditation may reduce stress-induced cortisol secretion, which I have covered earlier in this chapter. In fact, they report that this reduction in cortisol secretion could have neuroprotective effects, perhaps by elevating levels of BDNF. Meditation may also lower oxidative stress and have beneficial effects on lipid profiles, both of which could reduce the risk for cerebrovascular disease and age-related neurodegeneration. Further, the study asserts that meditation may strengthen neuronal circuits and enhance cognitive reserve capacity.

Besides the neuroprotective effect, BDNF plays a major role in energy homeostasis, the biological process through which cells balance energy production and expenditure. Energy homeostasis is critical for cell survival and proper functioning.

THE MEDITATION LANDSCAPE

If you want to look great and feel focused, calm, and energetic; and quiet inflammation; and bring your body into balance, you only have to invest 20 minutes a day meditating. When you think of meditation, you might visualize chanting, ascetic monks, but adopting a meditation practice should not be daunting. You can benefit significantly by dedicating less than a half hour a day to calmly limiting your thoughts and attention.

I want to familiarize you with the various options from which you can choose. The first overall category is guided or unguided meditation. If you have never meditated before, you might want to consider starting with guided meditation. A teacher takes you through the steps of the practice with guided meditation. The teacher leads you through a meditation technique and explains the process. You can choose to attend a class or a group meditation or take advantage of the many meditation programs available online. Countless guided meditations are available. You can experiment with several to find the right one for you. The other general category is unguided meditation, which is just as it sounds. This form of meditation is silent. You do the meditation on your own.

There are so many styles of meditation that you might be confused and feel intimidated before you begin. For the balance of this chapter, I will introduce you to a variety of meditation techniques and will later give you direction on how to perform a few basic ones.

In the broadest sense, meditation styles fall into three categories: open monitoring, focused attention, and self-transcending.

> **Open monitoring** involves observing awareness, which is the central theme of mindfulness meditation techniques, including walking meditation. It is a passive meditation. The practitioner notices thoughts and feelings without reacting to them. The term also applies to Vipassana, known as insight meditation.
>
> **Focused attention** is a form of meditation in which attention is kept on a specific thought or bodily process, such as a focus on breath or progressive body scanning. Devotional, Zen, visualization, and loving-kindness are a few styles of meditation that involve focused attention.
>
> **Self-transcendent** meditation focuses on a sound, word, or phrase. You focus on something unchanging. Transcendental meditation is the best-known practice of this type. Mantra and om meditation fall into this category as well.

I should add that yoga is a type of meditation. Because it involves physical poses, I will discuss the practice in more detail in chapter 12, on exercise. Yoga combines holding specific positions with breathing techniques and meditation principles. The posture-based practice aims for physical fitness, stress relief, and relaxation. Yoga calms the mind and strengthens the body.

In the interest of simplicity, we will take a look at four basic forms of meditation with instructions on the way to practice.

THE WAY TO MEDITATE

There are a number of rules you should follow before you meditate:

- Find a quiet place to practice to avoid distraction as you are learning. In time, you will be able to meditate anywhere.
- Do not meditate after meals unless you want to risk falling asleep.
- Try not to drink caffeinated beverages before meditating. You do not need extra stimulation when you are trying to relax.
- Start by meditating for 5 minutes. Gradually increase your meditation time to 20 minutes.
- Set a timer to avoid being distracted by wondering when the session will be over.

MINDFULNESS MEDITATION

With mindfulness meditation, you will focus your awareness on the present moment. Observe your breath, bodily sensations, emotions, thoughts, and where your attention is without being judgmental. Acknowledge what comes into your mind or intrudes from the environment without reacting to it. You are open, receptive, and nonjudgmental. You ground yourself in the present as it is.

The objective is not to clear your mind of thoughts or to achieve an out-of-body experience. Do not alter or detach from your thoughts. Pay attention to the present and notice when your mind wanders off. Be committed to staying in the now.

The simplest form of meditation is to focus on your breath to anchor you to the present moment. You might find yourself caught up in thoughts, emotions, sounds. Wherever your mind goes, come back to your next breath.

- Sit up straight in a comfortable chair with your hands in your lap.
- Close your eyes. Feel as if you are sinking into the chair.

- Take 2 or 3 diaphragmatic breaths. Notice your increased sense of calm.
- Begin to breathe naturally.
- Focus on your five senses—the sounds, scents, tactile feelings of the moment to ground yourself in the present.
- Turn your attention to the flow of your breath. Try to think the words "in" and "out" as you breathe.
- As thoughts and feelings surface, try to let them pass without reaction. Just observe the thoughts and feelings and let them go. Do not judge what comes into your mind.
- Return your attention to your breath. It might be helpful to label the thought "thinking" in your mind as you turn your focus to your breath.
- Return to the here and now. Shifting your awareness from thought to the experience of the present moment is the practice of meditation.

A SIMPLE CONVERSION TO MANTRA MEDITATION

If you are having difficulty concentrating, you might consider trying mantra meditation. The mantra becomes a tranquilizer that distracts from the flow of thoughts in your mind. For this reason, mantra meditation might be easier to learn.

A mantra is a word or a phrase that you find uplifting. There are many traditional mantras like "om" or "I am that I am." You might find it meaningful to have a personal mantra that represents your core values. A single word like "peace," "abundance," "calm," or "love" might work for you. A phrase can be an option—for example, "may I be happy," "may I be thankful," "may I be forgiving," "may I be loving," "may I love myself." You can change your mantra anytime to reflect your challenges or joys.

A simple adjustment to the mindful meditation directions is all that is necessary.

When thoughts or feelings surface:

- Turn your attention to the flow of your breath. Begin to repeat your mantra silently. Do not focus on the noises, thoughts, concerns, and feelings that flow through your mind.
- If you get caught up in a thought or distraction, observe it and push it away. Return to your mantra. Do not criticize yourself if you lose focus. Continue this way for the remainder of your session.

WALKING MEDITATION

If you have a problem sitting still, walking meditation might be the answer. Moving meditation, which can be practiced indoors or outside, can give you a needed break from sitting posture. This form of meditation is derived from Zen Buddhism, but there are many modern variations. As you walk slowly, you could notice the warmth of the sun, the rustling of the windblown leaves in the trees, or the sensation of your feet hitting the pavement or floor. You are aware of your surroundings and your place in them.

With walking meditation, you move in silence as you observe everything going on around you. The idea is to be present in the moment. This form of meditation is not restrictive. It can easily fit into your life. You could practice this form of meditation with any movement—gardening, washing dishes, or folding the laundry. Just stay focused on your immediate sensory experience.

A GUIDED SPIRITUAL MEDITATION

Spiritual meditation involves the desire to connect with something greater or deeper than the individual self, whether a higher power, the universe, God, or your most elevated self. The goal of spiritual meditation is awe, transcendence, a sense of harmonious unity, all of which raise us above daily troubles and concerns.

Father James, the patient whose case I have recounted, is one of the most exceptional examples of the transformative effects of meditation. He shared his practice with me, which I reproduce for you for your elucidation.

POSTURE

- Sit upright in a chair or on the edge of your bed with a straight spine and your chin parallel to the floor and slightly elevated. Your back should not touch the back of the chair. Rest your hands on your lap so that you are balanced and comfortable. This posture will help to engage your central nervous system.
- With your eyes closed, gently focus your attention on the front part of your brain or forehead, where decisions are made.
- Attune your heart and mind to the Source of All Life, all goodness, all love, all beauty, all truth—God. We can do this by turning our focus to the source of life within, and paying attention to the human energy field that surrounds us. This is like tuning a musical instrument, so that your being is on the same vibration or wavelength.

BREATHING

- The breath carries not only essential oxygen, but also refreshing intelligent life energy, which heals, perfects, and elevates our perception and love.
- Begin by making some space at the back of your throat by drawing your tongue back while breathing, opening the throat chakra or energy center. Even without being told to do this, people tend to find themselves doing it instinctively when meditating.
- In the correct posture and attunement, breathe through your nose, and on the in breath, direct that energy to every cell in your body, filling your body with life energy on a cellular level. Hold the top of the breath as you energize and attune your cells and then exhale. Repeat the process for 5 minutes.
- Next, direct the energy to your brain, filling and attuning every

cell. Balance the energy in the various parts of your brain. If you feel one side of your brain needs more energy, simply direct it there. You can make subtle movements of your jaw to help direct the energy.

- Bring the cells into attunement with the Creator God—the Source of Life itself. Let the life energy soothe any anxiety, troubling thoughts, worries, or harsh judgments you might have. When you've done this, move on to your emotions.
- Direct that energy to your emotional center. As you direct the energy there, it will feel as if a gentle, refreshing breeze is filling the caverns of sorrow, soothing and healing any hurts, wounds, or loneliness. Do not dwell on what caused the pain, only on its healing.
- Commune with the Source of Life.

PROGRESSIVE MUSCLE RELAXATION

Stress activates the entire musculoskeletal system for the fight-or-flight response. Increased muscle tension triggers a burst of activity in the sympathetic nervous system, which causes a constriction of blood vessels within the muscles and inflammation. Chronic and excessive tightening of the muscles puts the central nervous system into overdrive, which increases activity in the autonomic nervous, cardiovascular, and endocrine systems.

Progressive muscle relaxation involves tensing a set of muscles and then relaxing them. The technique works on the idea that once you can identify the sensation of tension, you can relax it away. The technique enables you to identify a specific tense place, and then you relax that spot. You observe the difference and apply it to all your muscle groups. Relaxing your muscles reduces the excitability of the sympathetic nervous system. You will relax your mind as you relax your muscles.

Progressive muscle relaxation does not require a big time investment. Two daily sessions of 5 minutes can have a significant relaxing effect.

GENERAL DIRECTIONS FOR PROGRESSIVE MUSCLE RELAXATION

POSTURE

- Practice progressive muscle relaxation in a warm, dry, quiet room. Muscles do not relax as efficiently at cooler temperatures.
- Do this technique before eating, so that your blood flow is not directed to your digestion.
- When you are first learning the technique, lie on the floor so that your muscles are completely supported, or use a reclining chair. As you get more proficient, you can do this exercise while sitting or standing.
- Let your arms and legs go, rotating out.
- Place your hands on your stomach or at your sides.
- To make yourself comfortable you might want to use a small pillow under your neck or knees.

WHAT TO DO

Progressive muscle relaxation deals with seventeen muscle groups.

- Focus first on your hands and arms, starting with your dominant hand.
- Then move to your face, neck, and down your body to your feet.
- The first step of the technique is to contract a muscle group, producing a great deal of tension.
- Release that tension all at once, which will cause the muscles to relax more deeply. You will relax as much as you tense, like the movement of a pendulum.

THE SCRIPT FOR PROGRESSIVE MUSCLE RELAXATION

- Take a deep breath and hold it before you tense.
- When you contract a muscle group, focus all your attention on those muscles.
- Tense the muscle groups with as much force as you can. Hold the contraction for 5 seconds.
- Notice the tightness and what tension feels like in those muscles.
- Let all the tension go.
- Notice the pleasurable sensation in those muscles. Breathe slowly for 30 to 40 seconds.
- Repeat the process with the same muscle group, then move on to the next part of your body.

HOW TO TENSE MUSCLE GROUPS IN ORDER OF ENGAGEMENT

Tense and relax these areas of the body in the following order:

RIGHT HAND AND FOREARM
If you are right-handed. Otherwise begin with your left side.

- Make a tight fist with your right hand, upper arm relaxed.

RIGHT UPPER ARM

- Press your right elbow down against the floor or chair.

LEFT HAND AND FOREARM

- Make a tight fist with your left hand, upper arm relaxed.

LEFT UPPER ARM

- Press your left elbow down against the floor or chair.

FOREHEAD

- Raise your eyebrows as high as possible.

UPPER CHEEKS AND NOSE

- Wrinkle your nose and squint your eyes.

LOWER FACE

- Clench your jaw and smirk.

NECK

- Try to raise and lower your chin at the same time.

SHOULDERS AND NECK

- Raise your shoulders as if trying to touch your ears.

CHEST, SHOULDERS, UPPER BACK

- Take a deep breath and pull your shoulder blades together.

ABDOMEN

- Try to push your stomach out and pull it in at the same time.

RIGHT THIGH

- Contract the large muscles on the front of your right leg and the smaller muscles underneath. Press your right heel down on the floor.

RIGHT CALF

- Point the toes of your right foot, then flex your foot back with your toes pointing toward your knee.

RIGHT FOOT

- Point the toes on your right foot, turn your foot in, and curl your toes gently.

LEFT THIGH

- Contract the large muscles on the front of your left leg and smaller muscles underneath. Press your left heel down on the floor.

LEFT CALF

- Point the toes of your left foot, then flex your foot back with your toes pointing toward your knee.

LEFT FOOT

- Point the toes of your left foot, turn your foot in, and curl your toes gently.

Going through the various parts of your body—tensing and relaxing—will help you to realize where tension is trapped in your body. You will feel lighter when you finish the series.

Spot Checks

You can do spot checks on your tension level during the day. If you have some hot spots, you can target them.

Neck and shoulders: Reduce tension or ache by lifting your shoulders up to your ears and relaxing them several times.

Core: If you hold tension in your core by holding your stomach muscles rigidly, contract those muscles even more tightly, pressing your lower back to the chair or the floor. If you are standing, tilt your pelvis forward and release your stomach muscles.

Shallow breathing: Press your shoulders back to expand your chest, and inhale deeply.

Furrowing brow: Raise your eyebrows as high as possible, then squint your eyes and wrinkle your nose.

Grinding teeth: Clench your jaw and smirk.

Doing the full progression will allow you to measure the level of relaxation you achieve in trouble spots in comparison with other areas. Progressive muscle relaxation will train you to melt tension from your body. When you can release tension, your muscles will stop sending stress signals to your brain, which will extinguish or diminish your body's stress response.

12

MOVEMENT AND
THE BEAUTY MOLECULE

ACCORDING TO THE WORLD HEALTH Organization, a sedentary lifestyle is among the ten leading causes of death and disability in the world. Being sedentary increases your risk of developing all causes of mortality. Inactivity doubles your chances of developing high blood pressure, cardiovascular disease, diabetes, and obesity, which is why being sedentary is now regarded as "the sitting disease."

Most people spend the majority of the day in their cars, buses, or trains, sitting in front of a computer, on Zoom calls, in restaurants, in front of a television. People even shop with a click of a mouse, never even leaving their chairs. American adults spend 55 to 70 percent of their time sitting or lying on a couch, ranging from 7.7 to 15 hours of waking time. When you count hours spent sleeping, say 7, being sedentary can add up to 22 hours a day. According to the Centers for Disease Control and Prevention, only 24.2 percent of adults in the United States meet the government's physical activity guidelines. It is time that we get out of those chairs and get moving.

The guidelines from the US Department of Health and Human Services recommend that adults should aim for:

- At least 150 minutes of moderate exercise a week. That is 30 minutes a day, 5 days a week.

- Muscle strengthening training, involving all major muscle groups, two times a week

The most common excuse for not exercising is a shortage of time. The recommended guidelines are not that difficult to achieve. The 30 minutes of exercise do not have to be sequential. You can choose to divide the time into 10-minute segments. You do not have to spend hours at the gym. You do not have to push yourself with a demanding regimen you know you will never keep. Walking is all you have to do to meet the movement guidelines. Building more movement into your life is essential if you want to stay healthy, live longer, and maintain youthful vitality and tone. You have to get on your feet and be more active.

My goal in this chapter is to make you aware of how easy it is to improve your life by making physical activity a part of it. The more energy you burn, the more energy you will have. You will tap into a deep reservoir of energy you did not know was there. An active life will not only make you look and feel better, but you will also experience a heightened sense of overall well-being.

THE BEAUTY MOLECULE AND EVERY MOVE YOU MAKE

Exercise results in increased secretion of the Beauty Molecule, acetylcholine, which is why physical exercise is one of the most important allies in the prevention of age-related disease.

Acetylcholine is fundamental to movement. Motor neurons begin the process by sending a message to the muscles to stimulate the contraction. Acetylcholine is released at the neuromuscular junction, which causes muscles to contract. Acetylcholine is the only neurotransmitter that is not removed from the nerve signaling junction by reuptake into the cell. Instead, acetylcholine is broken down into choline and acetic acid by the enzyme acetylcholinesterase.

Once you decide to move any muscle in your body, whether to type on the computer, take a step, or smile, a signal comes from the primary motor complex of your brain, travels down your spinal cord to the appropriate nerve exiting the spinal cord. That nerve transmits a message through a network of nerves to the muscle that will do the actual job. A bud at the end of the nerve holds a reservoir of neural chemicals, including acetylcholine.

To make a contraction, nerves send an electrical signal that stops a short distance away from the muscle. The gap just before contact is known as the neuromuscular junction. Acetylcholine is released from the bulb at this junction and locks onto receptors on the muscle, called nicotinic acetylcholine receptors, causing the muscle to contract. The receptor is called nicotinic because scientists noted that the receptors responded to nicotine.

STAND UP AND GET MOVING

Movement is another example of the inestimable importance of the Beauty Molecule and its manifold roles.

Making movement a regular part of your life should become a priority when you consider the substantial benefits of doing so. Being physically active has been shown to be a powerful strategy to control inflammation and to:

- **Elevate mood.** Exercise produces brain changes that regulate stress and anxiety, precursors for fight-or-flight and inflammation. Endorphins are produced by exercise, which relieves depression and lifts your spirits.
- **Increase metabolic rate.** When you exercise, you are burning more calories and need more fuel for your muscles.
- **Strengthen muscles and bones.** Exercise promotes production of the Beauty Molecule as it is released in the neuromuscular junction. As a result, AMPK is produced, which enables the muscles to absorb amino acids and become stronger.
- **Improve insulin sensitivity**

- **Lower blood pressure**
- **Balance blood lipids**
- **Improve sleep quality**
- **Increase blood flow to the brain,** which stimulates hormones that enhance neurogenesis. The hippocampus, the seat of memory, grows, which is a significant anti-aging effect.
- **Generate glowing, youthful skin.** Regular moderate exercise increases the production of antioxidants to protect the cells from oxidative stress. Those antioxidants prevent skin cell damage created by free radicals. The increased blood flow not only produces a glow, but also induces skin cell adaptations that can help delay the appearance of skin aging.
- **Reduce inflammation.** Exercising regularly is a strong anti-inflammatory and metabolism-improving strategy working through the release of acetylcholine, the Beauty Molecule, which you know is a powerful anti-inflammatory. When you exercise, your muscle cells release interleukin-6, a cytokine that is pro-inflammatory. However, it stimulates the muscle cells that also release the cytokine myokine, which has positive effects on the muscles. Myokines acts as an anti-inflammatory and growth factor and enhances physical fitness. Myokines lower levels of TNF-alpha, a protein that triggers inflammation. In addition, interleukin-6 inhibits the signaling effects of interleukin-1 beta, which produces inflammation, particularly to cells in the pancreas that produce insulin. The longer you work out, the more interleukin-6 is produced. One study showed that 30 minutes of exercise increased interleukin-6 levels fivefold.
- **Reduce abdominal fat,** also known as visceral fat, which is a source of inflammation. Abdominal fat is not only unsightly but also threatens good health. There are two types of fat: subcutaneous or under the skin, and visceral, found in the abdomen surrounding vital organs. Visceral fat is considered dangerous because it is metabolized by the liver, which turns it into blood cholesterol. Visceral fat also puts pressure on the heart and the arteries, increasing the chances of heart trouble. We refer to this type of fat

as "toxic fat," because it is a veritable factory of inflammatory chemicals, which increase the risk for heart disease, stroke, and diabetes.

- **Boost immune function.** A study showed that walking can protect you during cold and flu season. One study found that the participants who walked at least 20 minutes a day, 5 days a week, had 43 percent fewer sick days than those who exercised once a week or less. If the walkers got sick, the duration was shorter and the symptoms milder.
- **Ease joint pain.** Studies have found that walking reduces arthritis-related pain, particularly in the hips and knees. Walking 5 or 6 miles a week can prevent arthritis.
- **Suppress appetite** for an hour or so after exercise.
- **Counteract the effect of weight-promoting genes.** Harvard studied 32 obesity-promoting genes in more than 12,000 people to determine the extent to which the genes contributed to body weight. The expression of those genes were cut in half among the study participants who walked briskly for an hour a day.

If a medication were available that delivered all these results, most of us would be eager to take it. To enjoy these benefits, you have to get moving.

EXERCISE IN A BOTTLE

Although it seems there are no limits to all the benefits of exercise, the molecular and cellular mechanisms that mediate the metabolic advantages of physical activity remain unclear.

Research is being conducted to help us understand the mystery of the benefits of exercise, specifically research looking at changes in the blood. The goal is to identify the molecules that may increase in the blood after intense exercise. Researchers studied the metabolites of intense exercise and found a hybrid of two chemical compounds that naturally exist in the human body that united in a special chemical bond.

When we exercise intensely, we feel a burning sensation in our muscles, the result of the release of different chemicals. Scientists used to believe that burning sensation was caused by lactic acid, also known as lactate, a chemical your body produces when your cells break down carbohydrates for energy. Although the concentration of lactic acid in the blood does increase during exercise, contrary to belief, lactic acid does not cause muscle soreness. Microtears in the muscle are responsible for the burning pain. The healing of those microtears is how muscle tissue is built.

Lactic acid, produced from muscle contraction, attaches to an amino acid called phenylalanine. As you know, amino acids are the building blocks of proteins. Phenylalanine is found naturally at very high levels in certain foods like meats, eggs, and fish. After intense exercise in both humans and animals, the enzymatic condensation of lactate and phenylalanine creates the molecule N-Lactoylphenylalanine, called Lac-Phe, a blood-borne signaling metabolite that suppresses appetite and obesity. When administered to animals, Lac-Phe has some of the same effects as exercise, including appetite suppression, normalization of metabolism, and decreased body fat.

In the past, researchers believed that muscles produced lactic acid when they were low on oxygen, a condition known as anaerobic glycolysis. This supposition has proven incorrect. Lactic acid production actually takes place in the presence of oxygen, which is called aerobic glycolysis. Both the human and animal research now show that Lac-Phe, the combination of lactate and phenylalanine, affects the appetite. When administered as an exogenous substance rather than being produced by exercise, Lac-Phe suppresses the appetite in animal studies for up to 10 to 12 hours. In addition, Lac-Phe normalizes blood sugar, increases insulin sensitivity, and confers many of the same benefits as exercise. Scientists are excited about the possibilities of Lac-Phe's mimicking many of the effects of exercise. The question is: Can Lac-Phe be exercise in a bottle?

When researchers attempted to administer Lac-Phe orally in animal studies, they found that there was no effect on the suppression of appetite nor in body fat loss. The scientists concluded that the bond that holds the lactate and phenylalanine together breaks down in the digestive track.

Researchers are now searching for other ways to administer Lac-Phe that will effectively maintain its activity. As I read the studies, I recognized that Lac-Phe could be an ideal candidate for the transdermal drug delivery

(TDD) system, a method of delivering drugs by applying a formulation onto healthy skin. TDD had proven to be effective and protected a wide variety of molecules that could not be taken orally. I have undertaken my own studies of Lac-Phe delivery by TDD. In the interim, we need to continue to exercise in the proven way to decrease the risk for obesity, metabolic disease, and all-cause mortality.

Exercise is an effective intervention for obesity and cardiometabolic diseases, including cardiovascular disease and diabetes. Sprinting appears to be the most effective high-intensity exercise to raise levels of Lac-Phe, and resistance exercise also increased levels of Lac-Phe in the body.

GET A MOVE ON—STEP UP YOUR ACTIVITY

Movement and exercise are different. You need both to fight inflammation and raise your level of fitness. Movement, which I consider recreation, is about getting up from your chair and doing something you enjoy to renew yourself. Adding activity to your life does not have to be a grind. You could take your dog for a walk, work in the garden, dance to a playlist while you do housework, go for a bike ride, enjoy nature on a post-dinner walk.

Exercise is not limited just to jogging, calisthenics, or weight training. Scientists say that walking provides many of the same physical and mental benefits as aerobic exercise. The good news is that walking works for all fitness levels and is a form of exercise that is easy to maintain.

Many people are addicted to their trackers and try to reach the magic 10,000 steps a day. That number is arbitrary, but counting steps with a goal in mind is motivating. Being aware of the number of steps you take each day will tend to make you move more to get those steps in.

Forming a habit does not take long. It is the way to start breaking out of a sedentary lifestyle. If you commit to moving 20 minutes to a half hour 5 days a week, it will not be long until you feel better. Making simple physical activity a priority will give you renewed energy that will change your life.

If you are not accustomed to exercising, be easy on yourself. The best way to start is to make sure you stand every hour for 2 minutes or walk 20 steps when you get up. Add movement in small ways—for example, standing and pacing as you talk on the phone; hiding your remote control so you have to get up to change the channel or volume; standing for all or part of your commute if you take a bus, train, or subway, rather than curling up in a seat; listening to audiobooks or podcasts while standing to do a chore like folding laundry. You get the idea.

To help you fulfill the muscle strengthening training requirement, I am including a high-intensity resistance workout you can do at home with a miniloop in this chapter. The workout takes no more than 20 minutes. Regardless of your level of fitness, the 8 exercises work all the significant muscles groups. As you will see, this form of exercise grows with you as you become stronger.

HIGH-INTENSITY RESISTANCE WORKOUT

High-intensity training can apply to resistance training as well as cardio. Most people feel if they are not doing high-intensity interval training, they will not get results. The fact is resistance training is more efficient and creates less wear and tear on the joints than cardio.

Adam Zickerman, founder and managing director of Inform Fitness and author of the *New York Times* bestseller *The Power of Ten*, is a pioneer in this form of high-intensity exercise. He has this to say about the efficiency of high-intensity resistance training:

> Most fitness experts agree that the key to fitness and weight loss is resistance training. Only resistance training builds lean muscle mass, which not only makes you look better but also burns calories. Three extra pounds of lean muscles burn about ten thousand extra calories a month just to sustain itself. Having three extra pounds of muscle burns as many calories as running 25 miles a week without having to leave your couch.

If you are inactive, your muscles will stiffen and sag from the pull of gravity. Your body, including your face, will show signs of aging earlier if you are sedentary. No matter how old you are, regular exercise helps to preserve flexibility, lung capacity, joint mobility, and balance, along with the cosmetic benefits of increased muscle tone and elasticity. Building lean muscle mass has all those anti-aging benefits. Exercise will also improve your quality of life by giving you the muscle power to perform everyday acts as you age, allowing you to stay independent longer.

I have asked Adam to design an accessible high-intensity strength and conditioning program for *The Beauty Molecule.* You do not have to join a gym or run on a treadmill for hours to build muscle tissue. High-intensity resistance training will help you to raise your level of fitness and create more muscle mass in a lot less time than cardio. For optimal results, the full-body home workout designed for *The Beauty Molecule* should take you no more than 20 minutes, two times a week. The only equipment you will need is a set of resistance miniloops. You will want to increase the resistance of the loop you are using as you get stronger.

Adam explained to me that this strength and conditioning program focuses on slowing the pace of resistance training and fatiguing the muscles you are working. Rather than counting reps and sets, you repeat the exercise until the muscles you are using are exhausted and you cannot do another rep. That is the high-intensity part.

He emphasized that the best way to build muscle is to slow down the exercise and described how these exercises are performed. As you increase tension in the miniloop, count to 10 and pause for a moment. Then complete the movement by returning to the starting position as you count to 10 again. One rep lasts 20 seconds. The continuous motion during the exercise keeps the tension of the resistance in the muscle, not the joint.

Doing the exercises in a slow, controlled way protects your body and prevents injury. You impose force with speed, which you want to avoid doing. Force causes injury. By lowering the speed at which you do each exercise, you are making the workout safer. Your muscles are doing all the work. Not using momentum to help you accelerate your reps translates to ultimate efficiency. By slowing down, you are building muscles without the harmful side effects or risks associated with high-intensity workouts. There is no wear and tear on joints, ligaments, or other connective tissue.

Once the movement is complete you do it again without resting, then again until you can no longer move your muscles. You will know when you are at the point of exhaustion when your muscles burn and you shake. Muscle failure means working a muscle group until you have no more force left to give. You fight against the resistance, unable to move another inch. "Going for the burn" can be uncomfortable.

When you reach the point of muscle failure, count to 10 as you continue to push against the resistance, even though you cannot move the band a fraction of an inch. That final 10 seconds, once you pass the point of failure, is the payoff. It is when change happens.

As you do the exercises, he says it is important to breathe freely and consistently. People tend to hold their breath when exercising, which is to be avoided. Holding your breath can cause an exercise-induced headache. Holding your breath can raise your blood pressure and reduce the transport of oxygen in your body. When oxygen levels decrease, carbon dioxide accumulates in the body, making cells more excitable. The carbon dioxide crosses the blood-brain barrier, causing the respiratory drive to increase to restore the balance between oxygen and carbon dioxide. As you approach muscle fatigue, you will find yourself breathing heavily and quickly. Adam recommends panting in this final effort to increase your oxygen supply.

If you want results, you need to realize the level of intensity required. It is easy to stop short. Adam claims that most people work out at 80 percent. You have to repeat the exercise until the muscles you are working cannot move.

You may be happy to hear that after working out with this level of intensity, you have to let your muscles rest so that your body can respond and begin building muscle. Rest and recovery are significant aspects of the program. That is why you only need to do the workout twice a week, which fulfills the recommended strength training requirement. After each workout, you should rest your muscles for 3 or 4 days. Overdoing this workout is counterproductive. Exercise stimulates your body to become stronger by building muscle. Too much exercise gets in the way of the body's response. In the long term, high-intensity resistance training will allow you to maintain an exceptional level of strength and fitness for life.

The exercises in the workout are biomechanically correct, designed to get the most from each exercise without stressing the joint. Avoiding extreme ranges of motion while using force and resistance is the most efficient way to build muscle tissue without injury.

Adam told me he has witnessed his clients markedly increase their stamina and suggests that you might want to use a stopwatch or timer to see how long you are able to do an exercise before the muscles you are working are exhausted. It's a good way to measure your improvement over time.

Your level of fitness determines how long it will take you to reach muscle failure. When you feel as if the exercise is endless and you do your repeats with ease, it is time to change the level of resistance of the miniloop you are using. If it takes more than 2½ minutes to reach muscle exhaustion, it is time to change to a heavier, more challenging miniloop. If you reach muscle failure quickly, in less than 1¼ minutes, switch to a lighter miniloop. Your level of fitness will determine how long it will take you to reach muscle exhaustion. The challenge is exhaustion.

If you have not done high-intensity training before, start with the lightest level of resistance to get used to exercising in this way.

Remember to take it slow, and when you are ready to give up, don't. Just hold on another 10 seconds.

HIGH-INTENSITY RESISTANCE WORKOUT EXERCISES

Lateral Leg Lift

Target: hips, core

Muscles worked: glutes, abductors, abdominals, obliques

If you are worried about your balance, stand close to a wall or keep a hand on a wall.

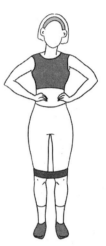

1. Step into the loop and bring it slightly above your knees.
2. With your hands at your chest or on your hips, shift your weight to your left leg and place your right foot lightly on the floor a few inches to the right, until there is tension in the band.
3. Squeeze your abs and tuck your pelvis as you slowly lift your right leg out to the side to the count of 10. Be sure to keep your knee straight and your hips square.
4. Lift your leg as high as you can with your foot flexed toward your knee. Be sure to stop lifting before you begin to arch your back. Hold for a moment.
5. Return your right foot slowly to the floor to the count of 10, keeping some tension in the loop. Be sure not to lean to the left. Keep your trunk steady.

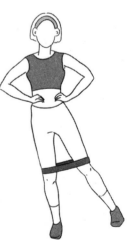

6. Repeat the leg lift until you feel you cannot do it again. Count slowly to 10 as you try to lift your leg.
7. Then repeat on the other side, lifting your left leg.

If you are having difficulty with this exercise, hold on to the back of a chair for balance and lift your leg a shorter distance.

If you want to be more challenged, hold for 4 counts at the top of the lift for each repetition.

Glute Bridge with Abduction

Target: hips and core
Muscles worked: gluteus maximus and medius, hip abductors, hamstrings, transverse abs

1. Lie on your back with your hands at your sides, palms facing down, bend your knees, and put your feet on the ground hip-width apart.

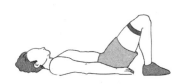

2. Put the loop around your thighs, a little above your knees.

3. Press your feet to the ground, squeeze your glutes and abs, and push through your heels to lift your hips to the count of 10. Make sure your body is a straight line from the shoulders to the knees.

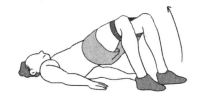

4. Squeeze your glutes and pull in your abs in this position and hold the position for a moment.

5. Then push your knees apart to the count of 10 so that you feel resistance in the band, while keeping your back straight.

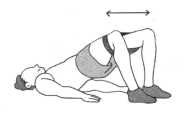

6. Pause for a moment before bringing your knees together slowly to the count of 10.

7. With control, lower your hips back to the floor to the count of 10.

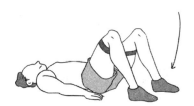

8. Repeat until muscle fatigue and count to 10 while trying to do another rep.

Russian Twist

Target: abdominals and shoulders
Muscles worked: obliques, rear and transverse abs, erector spinea, scapular muscles, latissimus dorsi

1. Sit on the floor with your feet together. Bend your knees. Place the loop below the center of your feet and pull it up far enough to take out the slack with your heels to the ground.
2. Elongate your spine and lean back enough to engage your core. Create a V shape with your torso and thighs—it should be a 45-degree angle. Make sure your spine is not rounded forward. Keep your abs contracted.
3. Slowly twist your torso to the right to the count of 10, while keeping your lower body stable. Rotate to the right as far as you can as you try to bring the band close to the floor.

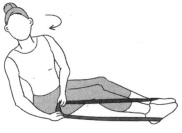

4. Return slowly to starting position to the count of 10.
5. Repeat until you cannot do another twist but continue to try to a count of 10.
6. Repeat twisting to the left.

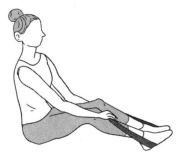

Once you have this down, you might want to make this exercise more challenging. Try raising your feet 2 or 3 inches off the floor and do the twists. This will work your core and shoulders more intensely.

Side Bends

Target: torso and obliques
Muscles worked: external and internal obliques, erector spinae, transverse and rear abs

1. Step inside the loop with your right foot and hold it with your right hand. Grasp the loop below the knee and place your left hand on your hip.
2. Stand straight and bend to the left as far as you can to the count of 10. Make sure to do this exercise slowly. If your movement is explosive and too fast, you can hurt your spine.
3. Slowly return to the starting position to a count of 10.
4. Repeat bending to the left until muscle exhaustion. Continue to try and count to 10 when you can no longer move.
5. Switch sides by stepping inside the band with your left foot, holding the loop with your left hand, and bending to your right to the count of 10.

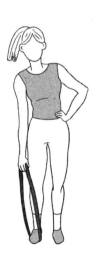 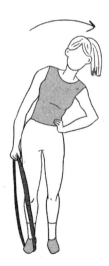

Seated Biceps Curl

Target: upper arm
Muscles worked: biceps and forearms, deltoids

1. Sit on a chair or bench with your feet wide apart. Step on the inside of the loop with your left foot and hold the other end with your left hand. You may need to lean forward slightly. Keep your core engaged and your back straight.
2. Rest your left elbow on your left thigh. Your right hand can rest on your thigh or by your side.
3. Start with your left arm at a 90-degree angle or greater. The band will be taut.
4. Pull your left hand toward your left shoulder to the count of 10, focusing on engaging your bicep and keeping your shoulder relaxed. Pause for a moment.
5. Return to the starting position with control to the count of 10.
6. Repeat until you no longer have the strength to pull your arm up. Keep trying to lift your arm and count to 10.
7. Switch sides with your right foot inside the band and your right arm holding the loop. Repeat the exercise with right left arm.

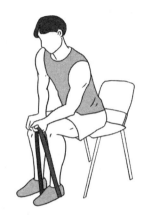

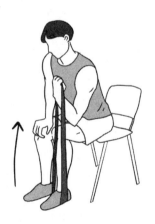

Single Arm Row

Target: upper back and rear shoulders
Muscles worked: lats, trapezius, rhomboids, rear deltoids, lower back, and biceps

1. Put your right hand on a table and loop the loop around your right thumb. Straighten your right arm. Hold the miniloop with your left hand.
2. Get into a staggered stance by putting your right foot forward.
3. Slowly pull back with your left arm with your elbow bent, squeezing the shoulder blade to the count of 10. Do not twist your upper body. Keep your back flat with your torso parallel to the floor.
4. Hold for a moment at the top, then return to starting position to a count of 10.
5. Repeat this action to muscle exhaustion. Keep trying to pull your arm back and count to 10.
6. Repeat with your left hand anchoring the loop, your left foot forward, and your right hand pulling back.

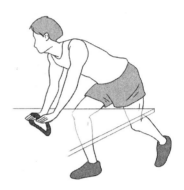

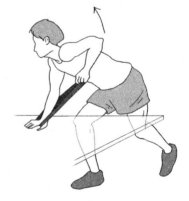

Lateral Arm Raise

Target: shoulders
Muscles worked: deltoids, trapezius

1. Hold the miniloop with both hands in front of you, with your arms down.
2. Keeping your arms straight, slowly raise your arms to the sides as far as you can go to a count of 10.
3. Slowly lower your arms to starting position, to a count of 10.
4. Repeat to muscle failure. Keep trying to lift your arms, pushing as hard as you can, and count to 10

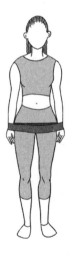
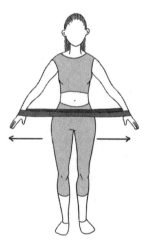

Shoulder Rotator Pull Apart

Target: chest and upper back
Muscles worked: rhomboids, rotator cuffs, rear deltoids, trapezius

1. Hold each end of the loop. Bend your arms to a 90-degree position.
2. Keeping your elbows at your sides, pull the loop apart as far as you can to the count of 10. Hold for a moment.
3. Return with control to starting position to a count of 10.
4. Repeat until muscle exhaustion, then continue to try to pull the ends of the loop apart to the count of 10.

Enjoy your increasing strength and sleeker silhouette.

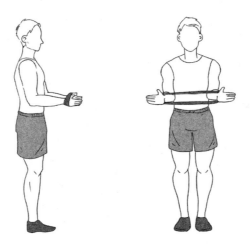

13

FEAST OR FAMINE

IN PART 1 OF *THE Beauty Molecule*, my focus was on *what* to eat to reduce inflammation. I turn my attention in this chapter to *when* to eat. Cycling between periods of eating and going without food, known as intermittent fasting, is an eating pattern rather than a diet. The focus is not on which foods to eat but when to eat them. The eating pattern involves restricting meals to a timed period, preferably not too late in the day to synchronize with your circadian rhythm. Intermittent fasting, also known as time-restricted eating, has become very popular today. I approached this technique with caution, because mainstream popularity is often accompanied by exaggerated benefits.

Most people try intermittent fasting for weight loss. The jury is still out on intermittent fasting as a method for that purpose. There is controversy about how effective this approach is for losing weight. Many experts report weight loss occurs simply because of the reduction in calories consumed. They contend that intermittent fasting is safe and effective, but no more effective than any other diet. The fact is that reducing caloric intake by 10 to 40 percent without causing malnutrition is the most effective way to extend your lifespan and your health span.

Although most of the research has been animal studies, the human studies are promising when it comes to weight loss. Dr. Mark Mattson, a senior investigator for the National Institute on Aging, reported a study of interest in a paper published in the journal *Free Radical Biology and Medicine*.

The subjects of the study were overweight adults with moderate asthma. They consumed 20 percent of their normal caloric intake on alternate days, a form of fasting I will explain later in this chapter. They lost 8 percent of their body weight in 8 weeks. The study found a decrease in markers of oxidative stress and inflammation, and an improvement of their asthma-related symptoms.

Flipping the switch between eating and fasting does more that help us to burn calories, which is why I am devoting a chapter to time-restricted eating. I will explore those benefits after considering the safety of time-restricted eating.

IS FASTING SAFE? ENSURING ADEQUATE NUTRIENT INTAKE

There are many benefits to fasting, which I describe in this chapter. However, my hesitation is that you will not be able to get enough nutrients in a very short window of time. It is essential that we get enough high-quality protein every day. As we learned, the days that we do not eat enough protein are the days in which aging is accelerated. Inadequate protein also exacerbates sarcopenia, which is the loss of muscle mass. We also want to ensure that we are eating plenty of fresh fruits and vegetables, also critical to the anti-inflammatory diet. Therefore, if you are going to fast, I strongly recommend that you limit it to a few days a week to make sure that you are getting enough vital protein and nutrients for optimum health.

You may be concerned that fasting is not good for you. The fact is that your body evolved to function without food for long periods. Our ancient ancestors were hunter-gatherers. They did not have three meals a day plus snacks. Feast or famine was the way they ate. The human body evolved to cope with an uncertain food supply and to thrive during times of food scarcity. Most if not all organ systems respond to fasting in ways that enable the body to tolerate or overcome the challenge of a fast.

Not everyone should try intermittent fasting. Those who should avoid the practice include:

- Pregnant or breastfeeding women
- People with eating disorders
- People who are underweight
- Children under eighteen
- Those who must take medication with food

FASTING AND METABOLIC SWITCHING

Normally your body uses glucose in your bloodstream, derived from carbohydrates you consume for energy. When there is more sugar in your bloodstream than you need, your liver stores the glucose. If your body is in a fasting state, metabolic changes occur. It takes 10 to 12 hours of fasting to use up calories in the bloodstream, and energy stored in the liver in the form of glycogen, before a metabolic shift occurs. Subsequently, your body produces less insulin because there are low levels of blood sugar circulating in your bloodstream.

Once the glucose in your bloodstream and liver is depleted, the body switches to fat burning for energy to compensate. This fat-burning state produces ketones for energy and homeostasis. Ketones act as an alternative fuel favored by the brain, and also preserve muscle mass. During a fasting period, the body adjusts hormone levels to make stored body fat more accessible, cells initiate repair processes, and the expression of genes change. The effect of this metabolic switching is what interests me. A study in the *New England Journal of Medicine* suggests that intermittent fasting leads to a longer life, leaner body, and sharper mind.

A TIMELINE OF FASTING EFFECTS ON THE BODY

Your body goes through four stages as you fast. What follows is an hour-by-hour account of the stages of physiological effects of fasting. The time is based on the last time you ate.

Phase 1: The Anabolic Stage

0–4 HOURS

- Body uses the energy from the food you just ate for energy and for cellular and tissue growth
- Pancreas secretes insulin to use the glucose in the bloodstream and store the excess in cells

Phase 2: The Catabolic Stage

From 4 to 16 hours of fasting is the breakdown phase, when the body uses stored nutrients. Glycogen stores are broken down and used for energy.

4–8 HOURS

- Blood sugars fall
- All food has left the stomach
- Insulin is no longer produced

12 HOURS

- Food consumed has been burned
- Digestive system goes to sleep
- Body begins healing process

- Human growth hormone begins to increase
- Glucagon is released to balance blood sugars by preventing blood sugars from dropping too low

14 HOURS

- Body has converted to using stored fat as energy
- Human growth hormone starts to increase dramatically

Phase 3: Fat-Burning Stage

The body begins to burn fat to meet energy demands because no glucose is available in the bloodstream.

16 HOURS

- Body starts to ramp up the fat burning
- mTOR, the growth regulator, goes down, which sets the stage for autophagy to take place

18 HOURS

- AMPK stimulates increased autophagy
- Human growth hormone starts to skyrocket

Phase 4: The Ketosis Stage

From 24 to 72 hours of fasting, the body has switched over to completely burning fat for energy, which produces ketones and boosts the benefits of the previous stages. The production of ketones is a built-in mechanism that ensures there is sufficient energy for the brain in times of food scarcity.

24 HOURS

- Autophagy begins
- Drains all glycogen stores
- Ketones are released into the bloodstream
- BDNF supports the growth of brain neurons

36 HOURS

- Autophagy increases 300 percent

48 HOURS

- Autophagy increases 30 percent more
- Immune system reset and regeneration
- Increased reduction in inflammation response

72+ HOURS

I do not recommend fasting this long unless your fast is supervised by a healthcare professional.

The body enters a deep state of ketosis. You are getting the benefits of weight loss, metabolic health, and longevity. Fasting for this amount of time has been shown to improve the body's response to toxin exposure and stress hormones.

- Liver produces IGF-1, a hormone involved in growth and development. Short time decreases in IGF-1, which occur in the previous stages, lowers oxidative stress.
- Autophagy maxes out

THE MANY BENEFITS
OF INTERMITTENT FASTING

There have been many studies of the biological effects of time-restricted eating. The studies have shown improvement in working memory in animals and verbal memory in adult humans. There is evidence that fasting can contribute to heart health, improving blood pressure and other heart-related measurements. A study of young men who fasted for 16 hours, whose eating period was between noon and 8 p.m., for 8 weeks showed fat loss while maintaining muscle mass. Studies have supported all the possible benefits of intermittent fasting:

- As long as bingeing is avoided in the eating period, the automatic reduction of caloric intake results in weight loss.
- Changes in hormones include the increase and release of the fat-burning hormone norepinephrine.
- Metabolic rate increases as much as 14 percent. Intermittent fasting changes both sides of the calorie equation: you eat fewer calories and burn more.
- Increased production of human growth hormone. Production of HGH decreases as you age. With fasting, HGH production can increase as much as fivefold, which benefits fat loss and muscle gain, reversing aging trends of increased fat storage and muscle loss.
- Improvement of insulin sensitivity. When you fast, the sugar levels in your bloodstream drop dramatically, which reduces insulin resistance.
- Reduces LDL cholesterol and blood triglyceride
- Fights inflammation. When your body senses famine, oxidative stress occurs, which triggers the production of antioxidants to protect your cells from free radicals.
- During fasting, cells are under mild stress, which is not necessarily bad. Much as with exercise, as long as you give your body

time to recover, which you do during the eating period, your cells become stronger.

- Stimulates mitophagy, the critical removal of defective mitochondria, and autophagy, which eliminates senescent cells
- Improves sleep as long as your eating period is not too late. Studies suggest that intermittent fasting during the day can strengthen and synchronize your circadian clock.
- Increases the brain hormone BDNF, which is believed to aid in the growth of new brain cells
- Increases NAD, the longevity coenzyme that affects metabolic health, DNA repair, and energy production
- Changes the epigenetics of genes related to longevity and disease protection

CATHERINE'S STORY: GIVING THANKS WHEN EVERY DAY BECOMES THANKSGIVING

It was a blustery April day as my dog Remy and I set out for our morning constitutional along Connecticut's rocky shoreline. Barking with excitement, she ran ahead to greet an old friend, a playful fox terrier named Rolly who belongs to our distant neighbors Catherine and Jack.

I had not seen Catherine in months; she and her husband, both architectural historians, had been away working on a project in Rhode Island. Their work was in high demand throughout New England. As Catherine approached, I tried to compose my features to not show the surprise I was experiencing on seeing her. Although she was recognizable, it was hard for me not to react to her dramatic transformation.

Catherine gave me a warm greeting and told me that she had been planning to give me a call. The dogs played in the water of the Sound while we caught up on the local news.

She asked me my professional opinion of the OMAD plan and added that there was no one whose opinion she valued more when it came to health.

She went on to tell me that the previous winter, her husband and part-ner had suffered a serious health scare that necessitated a trip to the hos-pital and a surgical procedure.

Catherine said she was happy to report that Jack was now fine. In fact, she said he was better than fine. They both regarded his hospitalization as a wake-up call that inspired Jack to start the one-meal-a-day program, and it had amazed her to see how rapidly he slimmed down. Her relief was obvious. She told me that she too needed to lose some serious weight but never thought she could stick to the program.

I have seen a great many benefits from different forms of fasting, and OMAD is no exception. I was eager to hear the details of Jack's experience with OMAD. Some experts insist on limiting the one meal to a 60-minute window and fasting the remaining 23 hours. Other proponents of OMAD are more liberal and expand the 1 hour of eating to 2 hours, which is 22 hours of fasting.

Jack's success was an inspiration for Catherine. She said he was much more stoic than she was and had fasted in the past for as long as 10 consec-utive days with nothing but water. But this was different. Jack had needed to lose weight and keep it off, which necessitated a major lifestyle change.

As she saw his weight drop, she was impressed by how rapidly he slimmed down. He lost more than 20 pounds and looked and felt really great.

Jack's remarkable success with OMAD inspired Catherine. She told me she had been tempted to give it a try.

Catherine said she was desperate and depressed because she thought it would be impossible for her to go that many hours without eating. The worst part was that she was not an overeater to begin with. Although she had avoided fats and sweets religiously, she still had gained a lot of weight. Life was just not fair.

Catherine did some research and learned that some experts believed that not eating for 22 or 23 hours would lead to serious hunger, lack of energy, fatigue, and uncontrollable craving. But her experience could not have been more different. For starters, she discovered how quickly a day goes by without having to think about food and what to eat next.

Luckily, she did not suffer from hunger pangs. To keep herself distracted, she made sure to stay busy as well as focused on a meal plan for dinner. In her mind, she was not fasting per se—just delaying the meal. After all, she said, perception is everything!

Rather than being fatigued, Catherine found that she had more energy, both physically and mentally. She used to experience tiredness after she ate breakfast. That problem had now been eliminated. Because she had seen how much and how quickly Jack's weight had dropped, she was ready and motivated. Catherine knew that she weighed too much, as none of her clothes were fitting. She was delighted to think that she could slim down just by delaying *when* she ate and not *what* she ate. The plan did not seem daunting. She did not have to give up eating altogether—OMAD is not that kind of fast. It worked for her.

Catherine discovered that having just one meal a day changed the entire dynamic around eating at their house. She and Jack would meticulously plan out their one meal with the same attention to detail they would devote to a special dinner party—even though it was a dinner party for two. That meal took on a new dimension. Every day became Thanksgiving, and their level of appreciation for nature's bounty was reborn. Instead of just grabbing something on the go, eating out of habit, or mindlessly putting food in their mouths to quell a few hunger pangs, they were both consciously choosing what they would eat for their one daily meal. Because they were truly hungry and knew it was their one and only meal of the day, making that meal as special and enjoyable as possible became vitally important.

As Catherine gleefully filled me in on her OMAD experience, I was not surprised to learn that she was now a firm adherent. Catherine could not get over the fact that she and Jack were able to enjoy all of their favorite foods—including a glass or two of red wine—and discover the next morning that she had lost a pound or two. Of course, she knew that any alcohol, even red wine, will slow down weight loss, because consuming alcohol interferes with fat metabolism. She knew that she had to be aware of that fact as she made her meal choices and set her weight loss goals.

Catherine admitted that her once-dreaded enemy, the digital scale, accurate to the ounce, had now become her best friend. She couldn't wait to get on it in the morning to see the results. It took her about 6 months on OMAD to lose more than 20 pounds.

Catherine said she genuinely believed that if people realized how easy and effective OMAD was, no other weight loss plan would remain in business. As long as you limit yourself to the one meal a day, you can eat whatever you want. Of course, she said, thanks to my influence they always made sure the emphasis was on fresh fruits and vegetables, good olive oil, and lots of healthy protein. Catherine and Jack both knew the importance of following the anti-inflammatory diet.

I was impressed by Catherine's enthusiasm as she detailed a day in the OMAD life. She not only looked great, but I could see that she was glowing with a healthy energy. Her skin had a radiance usually only seen on people much younger. Most of all, I could not help noticing how happy she was.

But Catherine had more newfound wisdom to share. She said that the OMAD plan had given her a wonderful sense of control over her life—a life in which almost a lifetime of dieting, denial, and major guilt if she ate anything deemed even the least bit fattening was now behind her.

Catherine reported that she could now enjoy the foods she had always denied herself, such as fine imported cheeses, organic whole milk yogurt made from milk that is classified as A2 for maximum digestibility, real butter from grass-fed cows, good-quality dark chocolate, nuts and fresh nut butters, even ice cream and cheesecake. She was ecstatic that she no longer had to deprive herself. A side benefit was that she and Jack had grown closer as they shared in their meal planning and preparation. What used to be a burden had become a joy.

Catherine also discovered that when it came to overeating, the real problem was the opposite. They now had to make sure they were eating enough. On the OMAD fast, they had to be certain they were getting enough high-quality protein and overall calories. They did not overeat, in spite of the long wait between meals. Overall, she had lost more than 22 pounds, and her weight had stabilized. She knew there were naysayers out there regarding OMAD, but it worked for her and Jack. They had never felt better.

Catherine shared another important benefit that had made her an adherent for the long term. She had not only more mental clarity, but also a much stronger feeling of well-being. She emphasized that she did not know if it was the relief of not having a 20-plus-pound millstone around her neck—and waist—that was responsible for her noticeably sunnier disposition and more cheerful attitude, which Jack also shared. They were happy to attribute their high spirits to another perk of OMAD.

Catherine's story is not unique. She has a small frame and is able to get the nutrition she needs with the one-meal-a-day plan. It can be more problematic for larger men, who need more protein and calories and tend to have larger muscles, especially if they are lifting weights or are very physically active. Our bodies are amazingly efficient. Eating once a day has a significantly positive influence on blood glucose levels and keeps the body in an anti-inflammatory state. For these reasons, different forms of intermittent fasting, including OMAD, offer much hope for physical and mental rejuvenation.

FASTING PREP

If you expect to suffer from skipping breakfast, severely reducing your caloric intake, or limiting food consumption to certain hours of the day, there is some good news. As you start intermittent fasting you might well experience side effects. Hunger, irritability, cravings, headaches, and fatigue are not uncommon. It can take 2 to 4 weeks before your body adjusts to your new eating schedule. The good news is that research subjects who stick with it feel better and more energetic than before.

During the fasting period you can drink an unlimited amount of water; green tea and herbal teas; coffee without milk, cream, or sugar; and zero-calorie sparkling waters. The tendency to binge can happen when you have not eaten anything for hours. During your eating period, avoid refined carbohydrates like flour and sugar; refined oils; too little protein, vegetables, and fruits. Eating this way will undo the health benefits you have gained from fasting. Stay with the anti-inflammatory diet, which will maximize the benefits of your fast.

MAKE IT EASY ON YOURSELF

There are some things you can do to help you to maintain your intermittent fasting regimen. If you want to stay on track, you might try to:

- **Stay hydrated.** You can drink an unlimited amount of water and calorie-free drinks while you are fasting. The fluids will fill you up and reduce any hunger pangs.
- **Choose nutrient-dense foods** rich in protein, fiber, and healthful fats along with vitamins and minerals.
- **Eat high-volume foods to fill up.** Eat raw vegetables, especially leafy greens, peppers, onions, cucumbers, zucchini, and celery; cruciferous vegetables like cauliflower, broccoli, brussels sprouts, cabbage; fruits like berries.
- **Go for high flavor.** Satisfying your tastebuds could help to reduce feelings of deprivation or hunger. Use garlic, herbs, spices, and vinegar to add a kick to what you eat.
- **Stop thinking about food.** If you are fasting for long periods, schedule distractions during that time. Go for a long walk, stream some TV shows, read a page-turner, get some chores done.
- **Take it easy.** Rest and relax if you can during a long fasting period. Indulge yourself—have a massage, take a nap, meditate to rise above any cravings.

PICK YOUR FAST

There are so many ways to fast effectively, I want to give you several options to help you find a method that works for you.

The possibilities include:

16/8 Fast

This is the simplest, most sustainable of the fasting options. Restrict your eating period to 8 hours. You would fast for 16 hours and have a daily eating window of 8 hours. That would mean skipping breakfast and restricting your eating to between 12 p.m. and 8 p.m. Or look at it this way: if you finish your last meal at 8 p.m., you will not eat until noon the next day. Some of you may already skip breakfast now and then. Others might appreciate not having to plan and prepare the meal. Of course, you can drink all the black coffee and tea you want.

12/12 or 14/10 Fast

If you find fasting for 16 hours difficult, do not get discouraged. You might try beginning with a less demanding 12/12 fast. You would eat between 8 a.m. and 8 p.m., giving yourself plenty of time for breakfast.

When you become accustomed to that schedule, you could shift to a 14/10 fast. You would restrict your eating to a period starting at 10 a.m. and ending at 8 p.m. You would still not have to wait for lunch to eat your first meal.

As you become accustomed to these schedules, you can progress to a 16/8 fast.

Eat-Stop-Eat Fast

With this type of fast you eat normally 5 or 6 days a week. Once or twice a week—days 2 and 5—you fast for 24 hours. That means not eating from dinner one night to the next. On the remaining 5 or 6 days a week, you can eat on your usual schedule. During the 24-hour fast, you can drink unlimited amounts of water, coffee, tea, and zero-calorie drinks.

5/2 Fast

On this fast, you consume only 500 to 600 calories on 2 nonconsecutive days and eat normally the other 5 days. On fasting days, the aim is to reduce calories to 25 percent of what you normally consume in a day. Again, your fast will have a greater effect if you eat an anti-inflammatory diet on the days you do eat.

Alternate-Day Fasting

Just as it sounds, you alternate a day fasting at 500 to 600 calories a day to one in which you have a 12-hour eating window. On days 2, 4, 6 you eat only 25 percent of your normal caloric consumption. On days 1, 3, 5, 7 you follow a 12/12 fast with an eating window of 8 a.m. to 8 p.m., for example.

OMAD (One Meal a Day)

This fast has become popular because the effects are quick and visible. The loss of body fat is evident early on. With OMAD, you consume all your calories in a single meal. You fast for 23 hours and eat for one. If you have dinner at 6 p.m. on one day you do not eat until 6 p.m. the next day.

People who try OMAD successfully report several benefits. Some people find it freeing not to have to think as much about food as they used to. They no longer have to figure out what to eat for breakfast or lunch.

OMAD saves a good deal of time. You only have to shop for and prepare one meal a day. By skipping 2 meals, you are regaining the time you would have spent eating. OMAD can increase productivity. Many people try OMAD when they are working on a big projects or have too much to do and do not want to break for meals.

OMAD fans say they experience increased energy, improved mood, improved concentration, and greater clarity of thinking.

MAKE IT WORK FOR YOU

If you have eaten dinner, then slept late, and skipped breakfast the next day, you have probably already fasted for 16 hours. If you find the 16/8 fast easy to do and feel good while fasting, you might want to try to move on to more advanced fasts: a longer fasting period and a shorter eating window, eat-stop-eat, alternate-day, or the 5/2 fast. You might want to ease into fasting by skipping meals now and then when you are not hungry.

You can change it up. You might try doing a 16/8 fast 6 days a week and OMAD 1 day, for example. You can change the length of your eating window when you want or need to. If you are invited to a late dinner after your eating window closes, just make the adjustment, and go back on schedule the next day. Experiment with the different approaches to find one that works for you and your schedule.

FAST-MIMICKING DIET

If fasting is not for you, you can try a diet designed to act like a fast. This diet was designed by Dr. Valter Longo, the director of the Longevity Institute at the University of Southern California. The diet requires you to fast for 5 consecutive days a month by reducing your caloric intake on those 5 days. To benefit from the fast-mimicking diet, the 5-day fast must be done for 3 consecutive months. The recommendations for calories and nutritional content are as follows:

Day 1

1,100 calories
11 percent protein
46 percent fat
43 percent carbohydrates

Days 2–5

725 calories
9 percent protein
44 percent fat
47 percent carbohydrates

Following this method of caloric restriction is said to result in weight loss; reduced belly fat; decreased bad cholesterol, blood sugar, inflammation, and blood pressure; slowing the aging process; and protecting against mental decline.

After returning to a normal diet after the 5-day fast, the body stays in the visceral fat-burning mode, probably because of epigenetic changes. Modifications in DNA and the proteins that bind DNA have been found to affect the marks associated with aging as well, which contributes to longevity.

14

TOPICALS

I WAS VERY EXCITED TO graduate medical school from the College of Human Medicine at Michigan State University in the spring of 1982. Armed with my newly minted diploma, I was looking forward to my pediatric internship at Yale New Haven Hospital in Connecticut.

I was not graduating with the class I had started with, because I had completed medical school in less than 3 years. I did not know anyone, but my family was there to cheer me on. My son, who was 6 at the time, sat on my lap throughout the entire ceremony. It was one of the most memorable days of my life. I had been headed to this destination since I was a young boy. Despite the many obstacles I had had to overcome on the road to that hard-won medical degree, I was grateful to be where I was.

I had 3 to 4 weeks to relax before my internship started on June 23, my birthday. I was happy to be at Yale School of Medicine/Yale New Haven Hospital, because their pediatrics program was one of the best in the country. I would be working under the chairman of the department of pediatrics, Dr. Howard Pearson, whose specialty was pediatric hematology/oncology. An extraordinary person and physician, Dr. Pearson had saved the lives of thousands of children during his brilliant career.

The evening before the first day of our internship, Dr. Pearson hosted a party for the interns at his home. Though I knew about his dedication to pediatrics, I was equally impressed by how congenial he was. We talked that night and throughout an incredibly hectic year.

Dr. Pearson was interested in sickle cell anemia and I, too, had been fascinated by this medical problem. I learned about sickle cell anemia while studying biochemistry. A sickle cell is a red blood cell that is deformed into an abnormal crescent shape. I was familiar with what is known as a sickle cell crisis. The crisis occurs when the sickle red blood cells block the small vessels that carry blood to bones. A sickle cell crisis can be the result of triggers that cause blood vessel constriction. Physical or psychological stress and even cold weather are triggers. The most notable symptom of sickle cell anemia is pain, particularly episodes of sudden pain. Fatigue is another common symptom, which results from anemia, a deficiency of healthy red blood cells. These symptoms indicate problems with circulation that can be life-threatening.

In my biochemistry studies, we discussed hemoglobin, the protein that carries oxygen to red blood cells. We learned that the level of oxygen could vary based on exercise or altitude. The biochemistry textbook I was using was written by a professor of cell biology at Stanford University School of Medicine, Dr. Lubert Stryer. The book was so well written I remembered every detail, including an understanding of proteins on the molecular level. The body could adapt to oxygen demand by creating a molecule called 2,3-diphosphoglycerate (DPG). Not only did this molecule act as a scavenger of free radicals, but 2,3-DPG could also increase the affinity of the hemoglobin for oxygen. For example, the red cells of an elite athlete would produce more 2,3-DPG to deliver more oxygen to the muscles.

If you were climbing a mountain, your body would begin producing 2,3-DPG in a matter of 2 or 3 days to provide the needed increase in oxygen to complete the climb. This occurs with anemia as well, because the condition leads to a decreased number of red blood cells, which means less oxygen is available in the body. With anemia, the body's mechanism goes to work to produce more 2,3-DPG to increase oxygen levels.

With sickle cell anemia, red blood cells sickle when they have given up their oxygen, which is known as deoxyhemoglobin. When this happens, the red blood cells become hard and sticky and take on the appearance of the C-shaped farm tool called a sickle. The blood becomes chronically low in oxygen saturation, which creates sickle cells that block blood flow to organs. The lack of oxygen-rich blood can damage nerves and organs, including the kidneys, liver, and spleen, and can be fatal.

Sickle red blood cells are not flexible, which leads to chronic hemolytic anemia and vaso-occlusive crises. Because the sickle cells die early, there is a constant shortage of red blood cells. When the sickle cells travel through small blood vessels, they get stuck and clog the blood flow, which can cause pain and serious health problems such as infection, acute chest syndrome, and stroke.

I had thought a lot about sickle cell anemia in medical school and had started to look for a way to inhibit the production of 2,3-DPG in those with sickle cell anemia. Studies have shown that there is a correlation between severity of anemia and increase of DPG oxygen affinity to hemoglobin concentration in sickle cell anemia. If I could find the right substance, more of the red blood cells would remain in the oxygenated form of hemoglobin, a state known as oxyhemoglobin. Hemoglobin has an iron center that acts as an oxygen transport protein in the red blood cells. The iron in the hemoglobin allows the red blood cells to pick up oxygen from the air we breathe and to deliver it everywhere in the body. The hemoglobin gives red blood cells their color. My goal was to find a substance that would inhibit the production of 2,3-DPG, allowing the cells to retain more oxygen and prevent the sickle cell crisis.

After scouring the literature, I came across an interesting and nontoxic substance known as glycolic acid, a type of alpha-hydroxy acid, that is derived from sugarcane. I learned about the molecule in my dermatology residency for a totally different reason. I spoke with Dr. Pearson about my idea of reducing 2,3-DPG levels by using hydroxy glycolic acid. He was interested, and wanted to hear more about the concept.

We performed a study in the lab in which we added hydroxy glycolic acid to red blood cells to see if the cells would retain more oxygen. We used the oxygen dissociation curve, a graph that is a vital tool for discovering how blood transports and releases oxygen. A rightward shift of the curve indicates that hemoglobin has a decreased affinity for oxygen, causing oxygen to unload from the cells. A shift to the left indicates increased hemoglobin affinity for oxygen and an increased reluctance to release oxygen. We hoped the curve would show a shift to the left, but we found that hydroxy glycolic acid did not penetrate the red blood cell membrane. We were not getting the effects of reducing 2,3-DPG. Although we were both disappointed by the outcome, I valued and enjoyed the time spent with Dr. Pearson.

When I completed my pediatric internship, I left Yale New Haven Hospital and Connecticut, moving on to the Department of Dermatology at Henry Ford Hospital in Michigan, one of the largest dermatology programs in the country. The number and diversity of the patients I would see offered unparalleled exposure to virtually every disease.

GLYCOLIC ACID

When I began reading the *Journal of the American Academy of Dermatology*, an article jumped out at me. Authored by renowned dermatologist Dr. Eugene Van Scott and dermatopharmacologist Dr. Ruey Yu, it focused on ichthyosis vulgaris. This skin disease causes an extremely dry, thick, and scaly skin, which often looks like fish scales. "Ichthyosis" is derived from the Greek word *ichthys*, meaning fish.

They found that applying glycolic acid, the smallest and most aggressive alpha-hydroxy acid, to the thickened skin loosened up the stratum corneum, the outermost layer of the skin. Normal skin, free from the brown, scaly patches, appeared from underneath the outer layer of skin. I was impressed with this major breakthrough. As I had during my pediatrics internship, I began studying glycolic acid again, but now for its therapeutic benefits for skin. I was intrigued by its possibilities as an important therapeutic agent for aging skin. My studies in pediatrics and sickle cell anemia made me well versed in the hydroxy acids. I was eager to explore this molecule and its potential effects in the aging process.

I scheduled a call with Dr. Eugene Van Scott and told him how much I appreciated his article on glycolic acid and its treatment of ichthyosis vulgaris. I told him that I felt this was the tip of the iceberg. I believed that glycolic acid in particular, and hydroxy acids in general, had a much broader application, especially in the area of aging skin. My studies indicated that glycolic acid is a powerful antioxidant and anti-inflammatory, both of which are important for preserving youthful skin. At the time, aging was far from the obsession it later became. The baby boom generation, to which I belong, was only in their thirties. The concept of aging was not on their radar screens . . . yet. In the years since, aging has become their obsession, generating countless industries and businesses worldwide. Boomers were open to many new experiences, but getting old gracefully was not one of them.

When I was deeply involved with glycolic acid during my pediatric residency, I realized it had a molecular structure similar to that of vitamin C. This led me to conclude that glycolic acid might also have antioxidant properties, which would greatly increase its beneficial activity.

While the incidence of ichthyosis vulgaris is somewhat rare, aging skin is a universal affliction that is more than just an aesthetic problem. As I explained earlier, aging skin and its inflammation component had been a huge interest of mine since histology courses in medical school and my experiences with the microscope.

I flew to Pennsylvania to meet with Dr. Van Scott and Dr. Yu to discuss my thoughts about the possibilities of the hydroxy acids for the treatment of aging skin. As we all know, glycolic acid went on to become one of the most popular and effective treatments for treating and preventing many of the hallmarks of aging skin.

In the course of the next decades, I proved my hypothesis of glycolic acid as an antioxidant and an anti-inflammatory by treating sunburn with topical glycolic acid. The redness disappeared more quickly in the treated areas. I published my article about the similarities between glycolic acid and vitamin C. As I continued my pioneering quest for treatments of aging skin, my focus was on topical anti-inflammatories like vitamin C.

VITAMIN C

My topical approach was to take the many antioxidants, which I had concluded were natural anti-inflammatories, and put them into a topical that could be applied directly to skin. This approach would treat the target organ. Instead of delivering antioxidants orally, which then had to circulate throughout the body and be distributed to all of the organs, I could concentrate solely on the skin by using topical agents.

One of the most important aspects of applying these antioxidant, anti-inflammatory molecules was to help them penetrate the skin, so that they could protect cells by mitigating the inflammatory process. This led me to explore a variety of molecules with structures that could provide protective activity, a quest that continues to this day. Because the skin acts as a barrier, I knew that if the molecule was water soluble it could not penetrate the skin very well. This point can be easily demonstrated by pouring water onto the skin of the back of your hand. The water will roll right off. If you take some oil and apply it to your skin, you will see that it is rapidly absorbed and has a moisturizing effect.

My thoughts turned to vitamin C, a well-known antioxidant. A huge fan of vitamin C, I had had the good fortune to speak twice with two-time Nobel Prize winner Linus Pauling, who advocated large amounts of vitamin C for treating common colds and even cancer. I felt strongly that vitamin C could be extremely beneficial to skin because it was essential to collagen production. I hypothesized that vitamin C could penetrate the skin, the target organ, and deliver powerful anti-inflammatory effects.

I based my theory on literature I had read during my pediatric internship at Yale about a study on children with asthma. The children were divided into two groups. In one group the participants were administered chewable vitamin C tablets. The other group of children received a placebo, a substance with no therapeutic effect used as a control in testing new drugs or other therapeutic substances. The children receiving vitamin C orally had a marked decrease of incidences of acute reactive airway disease, which is another way of describing an asthma attack. The children who received the placebo had no change in the incidence of the asthma attacks. I was impressed to learn that the children who took the vitamin C had 50 percent fewer attacks than the placebo group. This profound result was important to me because an asthma attack is a cascade of inflammatory events in the body. I had to conclude that vitamin C was a powerful anti-inflammatory. This information was of paramount importance when I began looking at topical application to the skin. My first inclination was to reach for vitamin C.

When vitamin C in the water-soluble form, called ascorbic acid, is mixed with iron in a solution in the laboratory, what is called a Fenton reaction then generates free radicals, specifically a powerfully toxic free radical known as the hydroxyl radical. Aging skin has higher amounts of iron available and can be more vulnerable to Fenton reactions. When water-soluble ascorbic acid is mixed with iron, a Fenton reaction produces inflammation—another reason to avoid topical ascorbic acid.

I knew that we did not want to put water-soluble ascorbic acid on the skin, because doing so could create a Fenton reaction, resulting in hydroxyl radicals and a burst of inflammation. When added to a topical formulation, ascorbic acid had difficulty penetrating the surface of the skin, a positive outcome considering that the Fenton reaction would cancel out any therapeutic effects of the vitamin C.

Ascorbic acid has other serious drawbacks when used as a topical ingredient, because ascorbic acid cannot protect cell membranes. The skin cannot maintain adequate levels of vitamin C when oxidative stress occurs, either from internal sources like poor diet and stress or from external sources like sunlight. Ascorbic acid also irritates the skin and is unstable when used in topical formulations because it oxidizes, turning bright yellow, and loses its potency.

I needed a different form of vitamin C for topical application—one that could penetrate the skin while not doing damage or creating inflammation via the Fenton reaction. I came across a molecule known as ascorbyl palmitate, also known as vitamin C ester, a fat-soluble form of this outstanding nutrient. Ascorbyl palmitate has been used as a preservative in foods. The FDA classified the vitamin as GRAS, which stands for "generally recognized as safe," a classification essential for any substance applied to the skin or to be taken internally. When I tested this fat-soluble form of vitamin C, I was delighted to find that it rapidly penetrated the skin and delivered visible benefits.

Ascorbyl palmitate is a unique form of vitamin C that contains palmitic acid. Fat soluble and highly skin compatible, this fatty acid allows the vitamin C molecule to penetrate the skin more deeply and increases the vitamin's stability so that it can deliver its therapeutic benefits. The palmitic fatty acid not only prevents the Fenton reaction, it also delivers powerful anti-inflammatory activity to counter the signs of aging.

I first studied the action of ascorbyl palmitate in the laboratory using a collagen sponge, which, just as it sounds, is a sponge imbued with collagen, used in wound healing and other biomedical functions. By using the sponge, I was able to observe the effects of ascorbyl palmitate activity compared to the ascorbic acid form of vitamin C. I saw much greater penetration of the ascorbyl palmitate and evidence of a marked increase in collagen production.

A SUPERIOR FORM OF VITAMIN C

My research with vitamin C ester, also known as ascorbyl palmitate, revealed that it was a superior form of vitamin C. Its properties were impressive. I discovered that fat-soluble vitamin C ester, unlike the ascorbic acid form, realizes this essential nutrient's full potential as an anti-aging agent. It displays greater antioxidant activity in our cells than ascorbic acid and performs this vital work at lower doses. Compared with ascorbic acid, vitamin C ester delivers 8 times higher levels in the skin than water-soluble vitamin C (ascorbic acid).

Because vitamin C ester can reside in the cells' fatty membranes, it continuously regenerates vitamin E, which is depleted by that fat-soluble antioxidant's ongoing fight against free radicals. Vitamin C ester possesses superior ability to stimulate growth of the fibroblasts that help to produce collagen and elastin, the strands of tissue that give the skin its strength and flexibility. In addition, vitamin C ester was more stable in topical solutions, maintaining its efficacy while delivering its incomparable benefits.

. . . .

Dry Skin and Inflammation

My next step was to test vitamin C ester on an extreme dry skin condition called asteatotic dermatitis, seen commonly on the lower extremities of older people in cold weather. The condition is characterized by dry, cracked, and scaling skin that is typically inflamed. My studies had indicated that inflammation was the underlying factor in dry skin. The more severe the dryness, the more inflammation was present. I conducted a study on asteatotic dermatitis by first applying a moisturizer base with the fat-soluble vitamin C on one leg and just the moisturizing base on the opposite leg. I found that the dryness resolved very quickly when the anti-inflammatory effect of vitamin C ester was added to the moisturizer.

I applied for a patent, which was granted to me quickly because of the efficacy of the studies and the uniqueness of the approach. I wanted to get the concept of treating the inflammation as a causative factor in dry skin at the forefront of effective treatments and, ideally, make the treatment available to the general public. To this end, I set up a meeting with a very large multinational company that manufactured and sold skin-care products worldwide. I was scheduled to deliver a lecture to many of their top Ph.D. scientists who worked in their renowned research and development department. I presented the concept of inflammation as an underlying cause of dry skin, a new and radical concept at the time. Although the lecture was well received, there was no apparent interest in the potential of my discovery. No one contacted me after the presentation to learn more or express interest in my findings. I wrote the experience off as a waste of time. I had lost an entire day of seeing patients in Connecticut by traveling to New Jersey for the presentation. Eventually I forgot all about it and continued my research and my busy life of seeing patients every day.

Fast-forward approximately six years. Out of the blue I received a call from an individual who identified himself as one of the research scientists who had heard my presentation. Deeply interested in my lecture on inflammation, dry skin, and ascorbyl palmitate, Chim Potini revealed that he had been following my research since my lecture 6 years prior. A cosmetic chemist, he had started his own company. He believed that he could help me with my formulations of the fat-soluble form of vitamin C.

I was delighted to hear from him and sent him some samples of the vitamin C ester formulations. When I received the samples he had created, I was very impressed. His formulas had significantly greater stability than what I could produce in my small laboratory. Ascorbyl palmitate, as well as many of the other substances I patented for use in topical formulas, can be very difficult to work with. Only an extremely talented and creative chemist would understand what I needed. As I discovered, much to my good fortune, Chim was an outstanding scientist. We shared the same kind of love and enthusiasm for science and the creative process. Chim intuitively understood the way I was thinking when I formulated the products. We worked successfully together for more than two decades.

I was using substances that had never been placed in topical products before. I did not use traditional cosmetic chemicals but always chose molecules that were food grade. I made this choice because the activity of the chemicals I was using was much more benign and more healthful for the skin. At the same time, the food-grade molecules were more compatible with many of the active ingredients I was using, such as vitamin C ester. Chim understood my philosophy as he formulated products. Our work together was seamless and produced great success for both our companies.

I marketed these unique products through my company, which at that time was known as NV Perricone M.D. Cosmeceuticals and is now called Perricone MD. These unique anti-inflammatory formulations with advanced penetration technology led to great international success for the company.

Chim and I had an exciting 20 years of creativity and unparalleled growth together. My journey to the New Jersey company for my initial presentation was not a waste. It was only a matter of time before my effort germinated and brought me an extraordinary friend and colleague along with it.

COLD PLASMA AND A DELIVERY SYSTEM

I learned an equally valuable lesson about what I considered my nonproductive efforts in an entirely different area of my research. Although my passion was medicine, I was also interested in physics. I was working on a separate project at that time, searching for methods of increasing the efficiency of jet turbine engines. My concept was to enhance the performance of current jet fuels by using electromagnetic energy.

After I started the patent process on these concepts, I was introduced to a scientist at one of the national laboratories in Los Alamos, New Mexico. The laboratory was one of several that had worked on the development of the atomic bomb during World War II. A diverse group of scientists at the lab were also studying ways of improving jet propulsion. They were interested in the work I was doing, and we signed an agreement called a CRADA, an acronym for cooperative research and development agreement.

I traveled back and forth to Los Alamos working on the concept of using plasma as a way of increasing the efficiency of jet thrust. Plasma, considered the fourth state of matter after solid, liquid, and gas, constitutes the majority of the visible universe. It is a hot soup of nuclei and free electrons, usually existing in an extreme temperature, about 6,000 degrees centigrade. We were working with a soup of oppositely charged particles that were permanently separated. We used a device called a dielectric barrier, which separated the electron from the nucleus of the atom without needing high temperatures to generate ions with electric charges distinct from neutral atoms. The cornerstone of this process lies in the dielectric barrier discharge technique, a principle I mastered during my tenure at Los Alamos. We were able to produce a plasma that was room temperature, rather than being hot. We called this cold plasma. The phenomenon of cold plasma presents a fascinating paradox: a state in which plasma can exist at atmospheric pressure and room temperature.

This two-year cooperative research and development project demanded diligence, perseverance, and a willingness to traverse the uncharted territories of plasma science. Although the initial objective to enhance engine efficiency did not yield the anticipated outcomes, our efforts were far from futile. The cold plasma research ushered in an era of discovery and innovation that transcended the original scope of the project, leading to groundbreaking applications in the realm of skin beauty and health. What seemed a waste of time and resources ended up helping me solve a problem I was having in creating my skin-care products.

Cold Plasma for Skin Beauty: From Engineering to Dermatology

The insights gained from the Los Alamos research paved the way for the conceptualization and creation of one of my most respected projects: a skin-care product that I called Cold Plasma. This product embodies the innovative use of cold plasma technology to facilitate the coexistence of active ingredients with varying electric charges within a single container, a feat achieved by employing phospholipids as insulators. Cold Plasma has since garnered acclaim for its ability to rejuvenate and repair skin, marking a significant milestone in the application of plasma technology beyond industrial uses.

The versatility of cold plasma extends to its efficacy in sterilizing medical equipment and cleansing wounds without inflicting damage to the surrounding tissue. By customizing cold plasma generators for dermatological use, it is possible to fine-tune energy levels to reap the benefits without harming the skin. Such devices, which are now a reality, offer a noninvasive method to enhance wound healing, combat cancer cells, and facilitate

cosmetic improvements by stimulating stem cells and promoting cell proliferation. This innovative approach not only revitalizes the skin's appearance
but also enhances its oxygenation and hydration, contributing to a youthful
and healthy glow.

Despite the Los Alamos project not fulfilling its original goal involving automotive and aerospace applications, the venture was far from a
setback. The work illuminated the potential of cold plasma in fields previously unimagined, as I found with my work in dermatology and skin care.
This experience underscored the essence of scientific exploration for me.
The path to discovery is replete with unexpected turns and serendipitous
outcomes.

As cold plasma technology continues to evolve, its application in dermatological practices promises to revolutionize skin care, offering new av-
enues for rejuvenation and healing. This chapter is more than a narrative
of technological advancement. It also is a testament to the resilience and
adaptability of scientific inquiry, highlighting how a detour in research
can lead to revolutionary applications that benefit humanity in unforeseen
ways.

ANOTHER DILEMMA SOLVED

Ever since I began working with ascorbyl palmitate, I had been faced with
a dilemma. I needed to create a carrier system that enabled me to put a variety of active ingredients into one jar for optimum efficacy. Each of these
ingredients had opposite electric charges. If placed together in a jar, the
molecules would clump together and precipitate, falling to the bottom. I
was simultaneously working on topical penetration enhancers. I had to ensure that the molecules of the ingredients could penetrate into all three levels of the skin—the epidermis, dermis, and hypodermis. Skin, the largest
organ of the body, covers the entire external surface.

This is an important focus of my ongoing research, because there
are many biologically active substances such as peptides that cannot be
taken orally because the digestive system will break them down, causing
them to lose their efficacy. Many of these active ingredients cannot be

injected because our endogenous enzyme systems produce esterases that destroy the biological activity of these molecules. To solve this dilemma, I continued my research. After months of work, I had a breakthrough with the carrier system I was looking for, which I described in chapter 8. Depending on the ratios of the active ingredients I used, this carrier could be sent to any depth of the skin and even into the bloodstream. The carrier would protect the active ingredients from being broken down by esterase. This unique carrier system was composed of a liquid crystal matrix.

All of my proprietary inventions were protected with multiple patents because there were so many efficacious applications. In addition to delivering substances to any portion of the skin or directly into the bloodstream, the liquid crystal could cross the blood-brain barrier. This delivery system protected the highly active and therapeutic molecules from breakdown in the bloodstream. Controlling depth penetration was critical. The application could be cosmetic, ensuring that the penetration was just into the surface of the skin; or, for medical applications, the ingredients could be delivered directly into the bloodstream in a matter of minutes.

Not until my work at Los Alamos was I able to solve the problem. The cold plasma delivery system took the topical application of nutrients to a new level of effectiveness. This carrier could not only act as a penetration enhancer but could also surround the various particles with opposite charges. The carrier insulated the particles, which allowed me to put them all in a jar. I was now able to formulate topical products with powerfully active, electrically charged ingredients into one jar, which could not be done before. I found that the products had much greater stability, which significantly increased their shelf life. I named my product Cold Plasma after the work we were doing at Los Alamos laboratories and patented this innovative concept. I was now able to deliver many active ingredients in one jar and keep them suspended in the delivery system rather than seeing them precipitate to the bottom. I finally had unlocked the secret to topicals that were effective and therapeutic on skin. Cold Plasma, a very important product for my company, continues to have strong sales to this day.

This revolutionary transdermal delivery system was so efficacious with so many applications that I started a second company to protect the many proprietary peptides and other therapeutic formulas, and to collect the many patents being issued under the transdermal umbrella. I called it Transdermal Biotechnology. By moving into medical as opposed to strictly cosmetic application, I was able to offer a much larger menu of therapeutics.

SPECIAL DELIVERY

I discovered the ability to protect and preserve delicate molecules that have a very short half-life by accident, as often happens in scientific labs. Many of our most fortuitous inventions have been discovered by "accident"! While I was conducting studies on a transdermal delivery system for insulin, one of the tubes was inadvertently left out in the laboratory for more than a year and a half at room temperature. Once placed in a solution, the insulin molecule quickly breaks down at room temperature, losing efficacy after 5 hours. This is why insulin must be kept refrigerated once it is put in solution for injection. When my lab techs brought me the tube of insulin, I decided to conduct a study to analyze what remained of the insulin after more than 18 months.

To my surprise, we found that the insulin had maintained 95 percent of its activity. This was after a year and a half at room temperature. This occurrence led me to put nitric oxide into the transdermal solution. Nitric oxide was designated as the molecule of the year in 1997. Three American scientists, Robert F. Furchgott, Louis J. Ignarro, and Ferid Murad, won the Nobel Prize for demonstrating its importance in medicine.

Nitric oxide dilates blood vessels, slows the deterioration of normal aging, and reduces our risk of cardiovascular disease and the decline of our brain function. The problem with nitric oxide is that it has an existence of only about 4 seconds because it reacts with water, oxygen, and nitrogen. Pharmaceutical companies are concentrating their research on finding a precursor that can be taken orally or intravenously, which will then convert to more nitric oxide production in the body.

Knowing how my transdermal solution had stabilized insulin, I began work in the laboratory to put nitric oxide into the transdermal. We found that it was very stable, even up to 6 months at room temperature, which is impressive given that its usual half-life, which is the time required for half the amount of a substance to be eliminated or disintegrated by natural processes, is seconds. Our next step was to apply the transdermal cream. When we did our studies with animals, the transdermal cream was very active in delivering the nitric oxide. The transdermal application increased blood flow, which was easily quantified by ultrasound.

ALPHA-LIPOIC ACID

In addition to vitamin C ester topicals, I was fascinated by an antioxidant called alpha-lipoic acid, which I discussed as a supplement in chapter 9. Most antioxidants fall into either the water-soluble category, like ascorbic acid, or the fat-soluble category, like vitamin E or vitamin C ester. Designated the universal antioxidant, alpha-lipoic acid is both water soluble and fat soluble. It can protect all portions of the cell, including the outer membrane, which is fat, and the interior of the cell, which is composed of an aqueous solution. Alpha-lipoic acid also had a great safety profile.

My studies of the use of topical alpha-lipoic acid showed it had positive effects when applied to skin. My technicians noted that there was a problem with alpha-lipoic acid because it gave off an odor in the jar. I discovered what was happening: Light, either sunlight or the light in the laboratory, was causing the molecule to break down. To solve this problem, I put the solution in dark brown pharmaceutical glass, which eliminated the odor problem. That brown glass became a hallmark for the Perricone brand of topicals.

The astounding clinical studies on the efficacy of alpha-lipoic acid inspired me to start a line of products based on the antioxidant. I found that when ascorbyl palmitate was added to the alpha-lipoic acid, there were profound therapeutic benefits. As my research continued, I came across the molecule DMAE, or dimethylaminoethanol. DMAE is not a direct precursor of choline, but optimizes the production of the Beauty Molecule, acetylcholine. When taken orally or applied topically, DMAE tends to increase levels of the neurotransmitter acetylcholine. Benefiting both the brain and the skin, DMAE is another example of the brain-beauty connection. DMAE is a powerful anti-inflammatory in its own right because it works on the cholinergic anti-inflammatory pathway.

As you have read in chapter 5, the chief neurotransmitter of the vagus nerve and the preganglionic nerves of the parasympathetic system is the Beauty Molecule, acetylcholine. Acetylcholine can bind to white blood cells with acetylcholine receptors as well as to the alpha-7 nicotinic receptor. When this nicotinic receptor is occupied by the acetylcholine molecule, the inflammatory reaction of white blood cells is turned down by reducing the level of the toxic cytokines. Three decades ago, when I was first using DMAE, many of these mechanisms of action had not been elucidated. Once the studies were done, a large multinational company wanted to license DMAE after they discovered the formula containing DMAE was less irritating than the control substance when testing for sensitivity and inflammation. DMAE exhibited many exceptional effects on skin including increased tone and tighter, smaller, more refined pores. Because of DMAE's powerful anti-inflammatory activity and ability to increase acetylcholine through the same pathway, the skin showed increased radiance. In addition, DMAE enhances the penetration of active molecules. When the Beauty Molecule is added to topical formulations, especially in conjunction with topical anti-inflammatories such as vitamin C ester, DMAE and alpha-lipoic acid, the results are very impressive.

Along with presenting the most up-to-date research on reducing inflammation, my goal in writing *The Beauty Molecule* has been to capture the excitement I experienced with the discoveries I have made and the scientific process that led me to my findings and their practical applications. I want to give you a sense of just how complex our bodies are, and how intricate the balance of interactions are that keep us healthy or lead to deterioration and aging. Most important, I hope to inspire you to lead an anti-inflammatory lifestyle, by providing you with accessible strategies to support the Beauty Molecule, protect and restore robust health, increase your longevity, keep you vital, and make you look as young and vibrant as you feel.

ACKNOWLEDGMENTS

Anne Sellaro deserves a special thank-you for her matchless writing skills, creativity, enthusiasm, and tireless support for more than two decades, enabling me to bring my message to millions of people worldwide.

Diane Reverand for her extraordinary editorial skills.

David Vigliano and the team at Vigliano Associates.

Elizabeth Beier and her wonderful team at St. Martin's Press, including Brigitte Dale, Erica Martirano, Brant Janeway, Jessica Zimmerman, Danielle Christopher, Nicola Ferguson, Susannah Noel, and Lizz Blaise.

INDEX

ABOUT THE AUTHOR

Dr. Nicholas Perricone is a physician, author, scientist, educator, and award-winning inventor. He is the founder of Perricone MD, a global cosmeceutical and nutraceutical company, the preeminent trusted lifestyle brand that pioneered the concept of youthful health and beauty based on his breakthrough technology. He has been issued 237 patents worldwide and has dozens of pending applications in the diverse areas of medicine, pharmacology, and aerospace. The recipient of the Eli Whitney Award presented by the Connecticut Intellectual Property Law Association, he is also the creator and host of a series of public television specials. Dr. Perricone is also the author of multiple #1 *New York Times* bestsellers, including *The Wrinkle Cure*, *The Perricone Prescription*, *The Perricone Promise*, and *Forever Young*. He is a Master of the American College of Nutrition, certified by the American Board of Dermatology, a Fellow of the New York Academy of Sciences, and a Fellow of the American Academy of Dermatology. Dr. Perricone is adjunct professor of medicine at the Michigan State University College of Human Medicine and has served as assistant clinical professor of dermatology at Yale School of Medicine. As would be expected from the father of the inflammation-aging connection, Dr. Perricone is now embracing the holistic work of the last two decades, expanding his reach with the formation of the Perricone Hydrogen Water Company. As an active scholar, Dr. Perricone is currently enrolled in the Yale School of Public Health Executive Master of Public Health program.